TWELVE STRIPES DEEP

TWELVE STRIPES DEEP

Copyright © 2022 by Mary G Bruno

All rights reserved.
Except for use in any review, the re-production or utilization of this work in whole or in part in any form by any electronic, mechanical or other means, now known or hereinafter invented, including xerography, photocopying and recording, or in any information storage or retrieval system, is forbidden without the written permission of the publisher.

Some names / characters have been changed.
Scanning, uploading, and electronic sharing of this book without the permission of the author is unlawful piracy and theft. Thank you for respecting this author's hard work and livelihood.

Cover Design and Interior Format
The Killion Group, Inc.

REL012130 RELIGION / Christian Living / Women's Interests
FAM021000 FAMILY & RELATIONSHIPS / Infertility
HEA024000 HEALTH & FITNESS / Women's Health

Praise For
Twelve Stripes Deep

"In *Twelve Stripes Deep* Mary brings a unique and needed voice to a rarely discussed topic. It is clear that she has sought the face of Christ in all of her sufferings. If you are feeling the nudge to read this book, do it!"
Christopher West, Th.D.
President, Theology of the Body Institute
Author of *Good News about Sex & Marriage*

"This book is so needed by so many people. Mary Bruno shares the intimate details of her struggles, yet writes with a light, accessible tone that makes you feel like you're at brunch with a friend. I have no doubt that many women – both those who have struggled with infertility and those who haven't – will feel less alone thanks to her words."
Jen Fulwiler
Standup comic and bestselling author of *Your Blue Flame*

"For any woman, or couple, that has experienced the difficulties of endometriosis – I highly recommend Twelve Stripes Deep. In this book, Mary bravely chronicles her own journey – a truly inspiring story of faithfulness, determination, and redemption."
Stephen J Hilgers
M.D., J.D., CFCMC, SPS, Dip. ABOG

"Mary's writing style is simply addicting. Her story telling is captivating and inspiring. This book tells a story that is best summarized as a dance between one's faith and one's suffering. I couldn't put it down."
Oscar Rivera
International speaker and rapper

"Mary's incredibly moving, witty, real story connects with the very heart of what it feels like to quietly suffer the cyclic trauma of unresolved and life-interrupting period pain. In her book, *Twelve Stripes Deep*, she recounts a decades-long journey of an unrelenting search for answers, provides practical pathways to physical, mental, and emotional wholeness, and offers the hope of solace and even unexpected blessings and victories along the way.

As a 7-year infertility survivor, I connected with Mary's story to the point of many tears, and highly recommend it to anyone who has struggled to be heard or to understand the possibility of rising to our own God-given greatness even in the midst of, or perhaps even because of, great suffering."
Anna Saucier
Women's health advocate, entrepreneur, and coach

"We had the privilege of mentoring Mary and Chris Bruno for their marriage in the Catholic Church. Their story and their long and painful struggle with infertility touches us in the deepest places. Mary's vulnerability and courage and Chris's passionate and supportive love for his bride come through on every page of Mary's book enti-

tled *Twelve Stripes Deep*. Because so many women are suffering under the weight of the cross of infertility, there is an urgent need for truthful, realistic yet hopeful words to be spoken and written to bring compassion and understanding into this area of marital struggle. Mary has provided a valuable resource for all who read it."
Lloyd and Jan Tate
Authors of "In Home Marriage Preparation"

"I have loved every paragraph I have read. I live and breathe this stuff every day - the complexity is hard to portray to those who don't dwell on this. Mary has opened her heart to talk about her journey to spiritual motherhood. She offers us the gift of her incredible wisdom and faith - a perspective only possible from enduring emotional, physical and spiritual pain and, ultimately, growth.

It would be nearly impossible for your doctor, close friend or counselor to delve as deep into the heartbreak of infertility as Mary does. She crumbles before you on the pages so you can experience her journey, then she leads the way to put the pieces back together - no matter the outcome.

This book is a must read for any Christian who is struggling or who knows someone struggling with the cross of infertility."
Naomi Whittaker
MD, OBGYN, CFCMC, FCI

"Infertility leaves countless women questioning their womanhood, the fruitfulness of their marriage, and their dreams of maternity. With honesty, authenticity, vulnerability, and courage, Mary Bruno offers a unique perspective into both the suffering and joy that an experience with infertility brings. Not only will this book encourage you as you navigate grief, surrender, and trust, but you will also grow in your understanding of the true meaning of maternity and fruitfulness. I wish I had this real and encouraging book years ago."

Chloe Langr
Author and host of the Letters to Women Podcast

"Mary's book is the anthem for change in women's health care. Through her own story, she shares the journey that many women face: undiagnosed reproductive health concerns being misunderstood or completely written off. Mary shares her story with clarity and thoughtfulness, bringing the reader along and, for many, probably identifying with the challenging twists and turns. I hope every woman reads this book because this is what fuels a revolution for better care & new feminism!"

Bridget Busacker
Founder of ManagingYourFertility.com

MARY BRUNO

With a foreword by Emily Frase of Total Whine

TWELVE STRIPES DEEP

How Infertility & Other Suffering Delivered My Greatest Joys

For Chris,
my best friend, whose love carries me through, and whose support of my dreams has allowed them to take flight

For Bella,
whom I cherish with all my heart, and with the hope of another child you can grow with - that you will always know how treasured, and fruitful, you are

and for those of You *who feel unseen...*

Contents

Foreword by Emily Frase..xi
Introduction..1

Chapter 1: Worst. Day. Ever..7
Chapter 2: Clean Up on Aisles One, Two, & Three...15
Chapter 3: Him..33
Chapter 4: Why Not Birth Control?............................41
Chapter 5: Don't Smite Pontius Pilate........................59
Chapter 6: My New Best Friend...................................67
Chapter 7: Why Not IVF?...76
Chapter 8: Spiritual Freaking Motherhood...............94
Chapter 9: Her...113
Chapter 10: ViCTRiX..133
Chapter 11: Them...148
Chapter 12: Suffering..163
Chapter 13: Sex & Marriage..176
Chapter 14: Hot Mess..189
Chapter 15: The Farewell Tour...................................197
Chapter 16: The Twelfth Stripe..................................219

Acknowledgements...234
Bibliography..238
Author Bio..241

x

Foreword

By Emily Frase

"Raise a glad cry, you barren one who never bore a child, break forth in jubilant song, you who have never been in labor, For more numerous are the children of the deserted wife than the children of her who has a husband, says the LORD."
Isaiah 54: 1 (NABRE)

I WAS INTRODUCED TO MARY VIA Marco Polo in 2018 when a mutual friend realized the conversation we were having about the Catholic meaning of sex and marriage would be greatly enhanced by the perspective she could offer as an infertile woman. I had no idea at the time that this meeting would blossom into a business partnership and deep friendship not a year later.

Aside from our both being from south Louisiana, there's very little Mary and I have in common. She's a melancholic, I'm a sanguine. She likes fruity cocktails, I have an affinity for Scotch neat. Crowds can zap her energy, while being the life of the party is my *raison de'terre*. She has an affinity for details and executing projects, while I just like coming up with ideas. She is permanently infertile, and I write this six months pregnant with my third child.

And yet, I can think of few people I have ever met who have taught me more about myself, what it means to suffer well, what it means to be seen, and most importantly, what it means to be a woman and a mother. This didn't come easily or naturally. As you may be able to imagine, the conversations between a fertile and infertile woman can traverse some difficult territory, and there have been *many* awkward and vulnerable conversations about our different experiences that were difficult to navigate at first. Thankfully, Mary is the type of person who leans into the discomfort, which inspired me to do the same, and that has served to expand our capacity for compassion.

Through these conversations, we discovered a key thing we do have in common, which is the understanding that women who struggle for any reason in the Catholic Church need spaces to share and process their struggles in order to live their faith as they were meant to. We both believe that the most powerful and effective way of creating that space is in sharing personal stories in an honest and vulnerable way. That is what Mary offers here to those who struggle with infertility.

There is such a sweet respite to be found in the Simon of Cyrenes or Veronicas (or Samwise Gamgees, for my nerds) who meet us on our walk to Calvary and assure us we aren't alone. With their presence, they comfort us, and even while they cannot take away our cross or may even be silent, they do what they can to carry us through it. It is rare for us to find or be these people because it can seem ineffectual or force us out of our comfort zone. However, it is precisely in this type of meeting and seeing that suffering has the power to become unifying, and so lose some of its unbearable weight.

In the past four years, Mary and I have both been awed by the number of times that what God taught us about his love and ourselves through our completely opposite fertility stories was the same. This is why Mary's book, while absolutely a much-needed gift to infertile women, is a gift to every woman who wishes to fully embrace what it means to be woman. Even for a fertile woman like me, Mary's story is an invitation to discover the gifts and talents that God has given us all, and to understand that, regardless of our family structure, all women are commanded to explore the limitless fruitfulness that is possible when we give God our "yes" in response to those gifts.

When Mary asked me to write the foreword for her book, she said, "All the books and talks out there for infertile women are from women who eventually had a child. I want to write a book for the woman who will never have a child, and let her know there is still hope." That is what you hold now. In sharing her own story, Mary invites women into a process where they can explore their femininity, womanhood and motherhood as the inherent gift it is, regardless of whether they ever produce a biological child. She doesn't do this with theological platitudes, but from her own heart. She illuminates the truth of the Catholic female identity in its fullness because she has labored to discover it.

Mary's story isn't a challenge to the Catholic understanding of womanhood and motherhood. Rather, her story shows us the narrow ways we often limit and confine the meaning of these states, which is not Catholic at all, but a reflection of our limited human understanding. Her story can remind us that the lives of the saints, though all expressions of virtue and striving for holiness, were lived in wildly different ways. This book is an invitation to see your life and your suffering, not as a curse or a cross to bear alone, but simply as a totally unique life with a unique call to love and to experience God.

What you hold in your hand is a beautiful, though perhaps less obvious and therefore less celebrated, response to God's command in Genesis for us to "be fruitful and multiply." Mary's pain of suffering through infertility mostly alone, surrounded not by her Simon or Veronica but instead by few people who could see her and her inherent goodness, has been the very thing that transformed her into a Simon or Veronica for you. As you read her story, you'll see that though she has not brought forth a biological child, she can still join in the life-giving words of Christ: "This is my body which is given up for you." That is the hope that her story offers, the hope that because of the God we serve, our pains and unfulfilled longings in time can become fruitful and multiply the love of God here on earth.

There isn't a set timeline by which you have to achieve that result, though. All that is required of you, as you will read in Mary's story, is a willingness to lean into the life God allows for you, and a seeking to learn what it is he wishes to teach you along the way.

Emily Frase is a south Louisiana native living in northern Virginia with her husband and two children. After receiving her bachelor's degree in architecture, she went on to work in the nonprofit world in DC for five years. She founded the blog totalwhine.com in 2018, where she shares her deep passion for living all aspects of the Catholic faith in a joyful and honest way, especially marriage, motherhood, NFP and fertility awareness. She is the co-founder and president of the nonprofit organization FAbM Base, a new fertility awareness database. She has been featured in FemCatholic, Theology of Home, Vigil Magazine, Letters to Women podcast, and The St. Philip Institute. Learn more about her work: totalwhine.com and fabmbase.com.

Introduction

THIS IS NOT YOUR TYPICAL infertility journey. It is a love story painted by three dramatic characters - God, suffering, and the joy that is only produced by willingly accepting both of them. "Willingly accept suffering? Excuse me, what?" you might be wondering. This may initially sound like a tall task, and it is, but it is also a transformative one. And I'm not referring to the suffering you can control. Any kind of pain that can be alleviated absolutely should be. I'm talking about stepping into and getting curious about life's perplexing grievances that we cannot seem to escape despite great efforts. Unfortunately, we all get plenty of opportunities to practice.

It takes no effort at all to imagine several examples of situations that can facilitate pain and grief in the human person. Look into the very heart of the one who reads these words. What has inspired you? What has saddened you? What has made you come alive? What has brought you to your knees? For me, it was infertility that crushed me in multiple different ways before I was rebuilt, eventually making great use of what ails me.

I hardly understood what it meant to suffer until I experienced the pain of infertility—an unexpected reality that hit me physically, spiritually, and emotionally. Nothing has been more intense, more unpredictable, and more enduring than my emotions—and I'm not the only one. According to *The psychological impact of infertility: a comparison with patients with other medical conditions*[1], a comparative study performed by Harvard Medical School, "The infertile women had global symptom scores equivalent to the cancer, cardiac rehabilitation and hypertension patients…" Reading the results of this study really put my pain into perspective and assured me that I wasn't crazy for feeling so low.

What has added to my perplexing emotions are the internal and external pressures of growing up in a beautiful Catholic culture which I love dearly, but whose church on earth has made it feel impossible for some to live up to the high expectations of "being fruitful and multiplying." Without the balance of reverencing all forms of new life *and* appreciating the gift of spiritual motherhood, it is easy for Catholic infertile women to feel broken and undervalued despite great efforts to be faithful. Catholic women are far from the only ones in pain. Infertility doesn't discriminate between different faith practices.

It's not uncommon to be greeted by the most adorable round bellies weekly in church, which serves as an abrasive reminder of this unexpected life situation. Being unable to get pregnant blindsided me, especially as I had few places to turn, whether due to lack of resources or friends who couldn't understand what I was going through. One in eight couples walk around carrying this often invisible weight, but few feel comfortable talking about it or have any idea how to carry the heavy load. Friends and family have a sincere desire to help, but often don't know how, *and* have their own heavy burdens to carry. Infertility is only one source of many that causes suffering. We live in a world that is full of it. No one is immune.

It is the natural human inclination to turn from suffering and attempt frantically to break free from it, but that's not what Christ did. Think about how incredibly powerful and life-giving His suffering was, considering the joy that it delivered with the Resurrection, and how it paved the way for the Holy Spirit to set the world on fire as the Apostles spread the good news throughout the world.

Christ could not have risen had He not died first.

Likewise, we rise with Him as we engage in the hard work of dying to our own desires. This has been my experience as I navigate the pain of infertility in all of its forms. Although it is countercultural, I have found that the healing response to suffering is more wholly realized when stepping into it with Him, rather than trying to escape it. This is hard for most of us to wrap our heads around.

I stumbled and fell on my face frequently as I tried to understand why a loving God would allow me to experience such deep pain as my husband and I simply desired to respond to the call to "...accept children lovingly from God and bring them up according to the law of Christ and His Church" as expressed in our wedding vows. I didn't immediately appreciate his methods, but His plan would unfold into something beautiful. Our adopted daughter is one of the many fruits of His genius plan.

There have been several life-giving revelations, lessons, and life-changing events that have taken place over the course of my seven plus years of experience. I begin Chapter One with one of the most significant, which presented me with my most difficult test in an advanced course of "learning how to love." When I wasn't *feeling* it, God handed me an important choice on a silver platter, and the decision I made that day would change the way I experience suffering. It changed the way I lived infertility, even at the varying depths I would get to know over the next several years. My prognosis and physical pain would increase in severity, but my joy and peace remain non-negotiable because I gave God my trust and He cannot be outdone in generosity.

I will probably always experience some pain coupled with the loss of that dream of feeling our baby kick in my belly. And that's okay. Grieving is a natural part of life, but it does *not* mean that I am wasted or doomed to unhappiness. It does not mean that I am stuck or alone. It doesn't even mean that I am not a mother. The fullness of motherhood is not defined by one's ability to bear children, but the extent to which we respond to our individual call to nurture new life in any of its forms. This is a profoundly healing realization for women with and without children.

The sources of suffering vary, but the response that restores hope is always the same and will unfold throughout the pages of this book. That healing response is painful, but voluntary; an act of the will that is within the reach of all of us. If it feels impossible for us as individuals, that's because it is––but God always accepts our invitation to move mountains. Infertility started out as an experience that would consistently rob my husband and I of peace and hope with each passing month, but it ended up delivering me some of my greatest joys. My despair has transformed into gratitude and *my* plans into great purpose. These are some of the possibilities that have been born from putting my Nikes back into the box, because eventually, running from suffering will become more exhausting than the suffering itself.

I may be biologically infertile, but my fruitfulness is bursting at the seams! I want to tell you about how I got here in this honest and hopeful account––twelve stripes deep into my experiences of infertility, suffering, and incredible joy.

CHAPTER 1

Worst. Day. Ever.

"In light of heaven, the worst suffering on earth will be seen to be no more serious than one night in an inconvenient hotel."
— *Saint Teresa of Avila*

IT WAS 2015 AND HOT outside when it should've been cool— welcome to New Orleans. I was still infertile. I worked as a home health Physical Therapist Assistant at the time and stopped home for lunch when I got a phone call that set one of my worst days ever into motion...

Up until those early years of marriage, life was going (surprisingly) exactly how I had planned, giving me a great illusion of control. You know how it goes—graduate college, get a big girl job, move out, get married, have ki— and that's where my plans came to a screeching halt. You can toss that idea of raising a basketball team out the window without the ability to bring even one player into the world. I slowly became aware of a jarring reality where the kids I was so sure I would have might never come into existence.

When most of us are young, we don't really *dream* of having kids. We discuss our future children as if they will definitely exist. "My daughter won't date until she's married" or "my son will never get hurt playing football because he will never play football" or "my daughter will be a dancer just like me—" rearrange the sentence structure and replace some of the words with your own and you've got yourself some very familiar predictions.

My children were going to play sports. Dressing up and princess movies were moderately entertaining to me as a child, but I *lived* for playing outside with the older kids and just about any kind of ball. I used the basketball analogy because I have always loved to play sports. I started out with gymnastics, then added swimming and cabbage ball (something I realized later was only a New Orleans area tradition–look it up!), then track and field, and my favorite–volleyball. Eventually basketball and softball would be added to the mix. The highlight of my high school years was playing competitive sports, a combination of both challenging and rewarding experiences with teammates that made me a better, and pretty coordinated, person. I considered college ball, but wasn't brave enough to try out.

Athleticism is something I had in common with the four ex-boyfriends who would each play a unique role in preparing me for what was headed my way. Eventually, I married myself a good Catholic man who is better at basketball than I am. He will never admit it, but the talent tables are turned on the volleyball court where I destroy him (insert evil laugh). So, when I imagined the children we would definitely and without question have one day, I could not wait to witness the amazing results of the combination of our athletic genes. But evidently, God had other plans.

There *was* reason to believe we would have trouble achieving pregnancy before we hopped onto the proverbial marriage bed, but I was one of those blissfully ignorant

people who assumed infertility would never affect them because
A. Catholics have babies and
B. Catholics have babies.

And I was a good Catholic girl. Of course, core Catholic beliefs do not suggest that one must have children to be valued or virtuous, but this is a message that I have found to be conveyed often, whether intentional or not. Regardless, the desire for motherhood was strong. And even though there was plenty of research proving that my diagnosis was likely to be an issue for us staring me in the face, I pretty much laughed right back in *its* face. It was like a staring contest that I would learn to lose—frequently, and with a lot of ugly crying.

The absence of a pregnancy was *not* the only thing holding me back from functioning as a normal human being for some period of time. The discomfort–ok, straight up agony–associated with my severe stage four & twelve-year-late diagnosis of endometriosis has changed me. Pain takes on a variety of forms: emotional, psychological, spiritual, and most certainly physical. I would learn to live my life planned around the monthly visitor which would regularly confine me to my bed, and random pain that would ultimately leave me at its mercy on days that could not be predicted. This added insult to the injury of infertility.

I learned to expect the physical pain, but I did not expect life after marriage to look so differently than those around me. I really hadn't heard anyone talk about or experience infertility, so I took for granted that pregnancy *just happens* because that was all I witnessed. I remember thinking we were *certainly* pregnant after our wedding night because sex makes babies, right? But I was not. Weeks, months, then years passed, and panic continued to creep in while every sense of control slowly bowed out. It just wasn't happening.

Navigating the early seasons of consistently failing at getting pregnant was strange and embarrassing. You feel every possible symptom or unusual feeling, then google to "confirm pregnancy." I have personally negatively identified all things from a head cold to a sore right calf (not even joking) to mean a baby was growing in my belly. It is amazing how many times you can be wrong, yet continue to be surprised when it happens again. I remember getting very familiar with a definition of the word "insanity," meaning *to continue doing the same thing over and over again and expecting different results.* I felt strong for a while, but the steady disappointment was weakening me. My perfectly-planned life sequence was undergoing massive reconstructive surgery before my eyes.

P+16

On my worst day ever, we had been trying for about two and a half years and could've filled a landfill with the amount of pregnancy tests I had taken. Nevertheless, p+16 somehow rolled around again and I was prepared to waste another one. Just to make sure we are all speaking the same language, I will give you some context.

"P" stands for "peak day," which is the day most closely associated with ovulation (when a woman's egg is released). After ovulation, a "corpus luteum" forms from the follicle that released the egg and begins to produce the progesterone hormone.

This hormone keeps the period away as long as it's being produced in anticipation of a pregnancy each month. It secretes a nutritious fluid within the uterus, during what is now called the "luteal phase," to prepare for and sustain implantation of a newly conceived embryo. If pregnancy is achieved, progesterone increases even more. According to the research of Dr. Thomas Hilgers, co-creator of the Creighton Model FertilityCare System, a healthy luteal phase lasts between eight to sixteen days, so if a period doesn't start by sixteen days after the peak day, there is a good chance that you're pregnant (that is, if the woman had sex on a day of fertility).

I rarely made it to P+16, so that alone was reason to celebrate! But because of the dysfunction of my system, my luteal phase was more likely to last that long for reasons other than pregnancy. It was a horrible trick my body would play on me from time to time but still, I was hopeful. And for the first time ever, I saw two little lines in the test window instead of one! It was faint, but it was there!

Dumbfounded, and still guarding my heart, I tried to reserve my emotions for the confirmation of a blood test—which meant I had to wait a whole day. But I was sure that *this month* would be different than the others. After the longest twenty-four hours of my life, I got that much anticipated phone call from my doctor confirming that there was *no baby* in my belly. It had been my first (and only) **false positive**—a different result than the others, but not in the way we had hoped.

What felt like cycle to cycle rejection had been enough to wear me out, but this was a much steeper emotional drop within twenty-four hours that I was not prepared for. Not only could I *not* get pregnant, but I couldn't get the assurance of a negative test? Are you freaking serious, God?

I was mad and knew exactly who to blame.

I had had *enough.* My first reaction was to slowly turn and fix my beady-eyed death-glare on the Crucifix that hung above the door in our room while three words scrolled through my mind, underlined in red and written in one of those angry bold fonts:

"How could You?"

Tough Love
What happened next is *not* the heroic love story you might want or expect, but it is a love story. I was about to get a crash course in "Depths of Love" that I didn't realize I signed up for. I had always desired to know God more intimately, like most of us claim, but wasn't easily willing to give him my unconditional trust when it got so hard. And even as I gazed at him with blame, I begged for comfort.

But He withheld it.

I felt betrayed. I had been a naive cradle Catholic who never understood how someone could lose their faith. It was the only day I ever truly feared that God wasn't real. Sitting alone in my bedroom, an unknown amount of time passed as I explored the darkness and finally found nine words directed towards me:

"You claim to love Me. Do you mean it?"

I searched myself for an honest answer. I recognized how frequently and easily I either internally or verbally expressed my love for Him over the years. I grew up in a devout Catholic family, went to Catholic schools, participated in youth groups, became a youth minister at one point, received all the Sacraments, did all the things, you know the drill...

So, it was true that I claimed it. Yet, there I was in a puddle of desperation and sorrow questioning *His* love because I wasn't getting what I wanted. For me, it really was that simple.

Then the tough love followed:

"Then love me."

This was a truth bomb I was in desperate need of. He desired for me to choose Him even when I was hurting badly; even when I didn't agree with His will and didn't *feel* His presence. He wanted me to choose Him for who He is and not what He can give me – or for what He can take away.

I had become lost in my "need" for a pregnancy, but what I *actually* needed was Him—genuinely and without excuse. No one would blame any infertile woman for feeling such deep sorrow, but I wasn't *just* feeling sad. I was questioning God's love for me at the very least... and His existence at most. But only He could fill the emptiness Chris and I felt, and it was time for me to take an honest interest in my Creator's desires for a change.

The excitement of a pregnancy announcement *and a pregnancy* will fade. The joy of selfless, unconditional love will not; the joy that only Christ can provide *will not*! Love isn't a feeling that can change with the direction of the wind. It is an act of the will—a free choice that we make or we don't, even when it doesn't feel good and even when we don't get what we want. Making the choice daily is the only way we experience lasting relationships—even the ones that transcend time and space.

"Love is not a feeling. It's a choice," is something my dad would always say to my siblings and I growing up—especially in light of any pending teenage suitors. Now, I'm not saying that message didn't take about ten years or so to sink in, but it is absolutely one of the best factual tidbits we can gift little humans with. Whether or not the wonderful excitement of a budding relationship with God, a friend, or a member of the opposite sex is present, and even when the connection isn't permanent, understanding love as a choice is imperative.

That four letter word often results in good *feelings*, but the actions it requires can be very difficult; even downright painful. Knowledge of love's true definition teaches us how we deserve to be treated *and* how to treat others. Don't you wish that would be spray painted across the side of every high school and locker room in America?

If there's anything else that can bring on a *"worst day ever"* kind of feeling, it's the break-up of young love. Those teenage suitors my dad was preparing me for would grow up to be my young adult boyfriends. They would give me my first few lessons in this *school of love*, shaping my expectations, sharpening my faith, and even delivering a shock, or three, thickening my skin like only ex-boyfriends can.

CHAPTER 2

Clean Up on Aisles One, Two, & Three

"Everything comes from love, all is ordained for the salvation of man, God does nothing without this goal in mind."
— *Saint Catherine of Siena*

M Y WORST DAY EVER DIDN'T bring me my only heartbreak–not even the only heartbreak that wiped the floor with me–just the only one that made me question the existence of God. Before every girl dreams of her bouncing baby girl or boy, she dreams of her knight in shining armor. Not unlike my path to purpose, my guy did not come in the way I originally expected, and thank God for that! If things had worked out the way *I* had planned, I never would've met the man who draws me expensive bubble baths when I'm at my worst (don't worry, I'll explain later).

My first experiences of deep emotional pain came as the result of a few breakups. God used each failed romantic relationship to teach me about love and friendship with Him. My parents gave me a solid Catholic foundation, but it was through my relationships, and their subsequent demise, that I got to know the person of Christ. That brings us to the four prerequisites that helped to prepare me for what would become my greatest crosses and greatest joys: Nate, Dominic, Jake, and Miles. No, these are not their real names.

Nate
I had three boyfriends in high school and none of them lasted much more than a month. I unintentionally took my teen romances a little too seriously even before I started to care that the purpose of dating was to discern marriage. I even broke up with one of them because I somehow feared that being in a relationship meant that I would have to marry him one day. That's a little embarrassing to admit, but it illustrates how seriously I took dating. I couldn't have dated *just for fun* if I tried. There was some internal acknowledgement that I was searching for my future husband.

Needless to say, my first *real* relationship left a dent. I was working in the barbecue restaurant at Zephyrs Stadium (now called *"New Orleans Baby Cakes,"* a strange downgrade for a team name if you ask me), the home of the New Orleans AAA baseball team, when I spotted their super cute mascot with an athletic build walking by as we prepped for the game. I had also heard that he was very much into his faith. I knew I was in trouble.

Whether we say it out loud or not, every girl has a list of non-negotiable qualities for hopeful suitors. Top three for me and not listed in any particular order were:
1) Easy on the eyes
2) Athletic
3) In love with Jesus

Nate and I were both attending the University of New Orleans (UNO) at the time and he checked all three boxes, but it was his passion for his faith that was especially attractive to me. I was active in my youth group all throughout high school, but I had never met a guy that was making Jesus a priority in life like he was. The main problem with the trajectory of our relationship was that, as on fire for Jesus as he was, he did not believe in some of the things that I consider to be the most beautiful and core aspects of my faith: the Sacraments, devotion to the Blessed Mother, existence of purgatory, etc. You guessed it. He referred to himself as a "non-denominational Christian" and he wore it very well.

The Catholic faith I witnessed had incredible dimensions of piety and practice, but lacked a certain amount of zeal for a personal relationship with Christ and service to neighbor. In reality, authentic Catholicism radiates love of God and love of neighbor, but it is no secret that our Protestant brothers and sisters thrive in many areas where some Catholics, myself included, should take note and adjust accordingly.

Nate brought me into the city to serve the poor, he consistently got people together to pray, hosted bible studies and praise and worship both on and off campus, he worked his faith beautifully into conversations with anyone, regardless of who they were, organized free breakfasts, and even encouraged me to start a Catholic group on campus, which I did. There are many Catholics who are just as excellent at engaging with the community as he was, but what I witnessed from him was a deeper and more "hands-on" dimension of loving your neighbor than I was personally used to.

I learned a lot from him and soon realized how little I knew about my own faith. I will never forget that one day when we were riding in his car and listening to Chris Tomlin's "Your Grace is Enough" when I asked him, "Is this what I believe as a Catholic?" He gave me an incredibly confused glance and said, "Yyyes." (Is it possible for me to embarrass myself anymore?) I knew what the obvious differences between our beliefs were, but I was unable to articulate my faith at a very fundamental level. Thankfully, I was a deeply convicted Catholic even if I didn't completely understand why yet. So, instead of simply ditching the Sacraments, I used this as an opportunity to get curious and understand *why* we believe what we do.

I used to refer to my parents as the Pope's best friends because they have always known almost every specific detail of Church teaching and exactly where to find it. So, I knew exactly who to turn to. My dad's book shelves are still graced with a wide assortment of the colorful book cover variations of Peter Kreeft, Brant Pitre, John Bergsma, commentaries on the entire Bible, a range of encyclicals, apologetics, writings of Popes and Saints, and much more. There was no Bon Jovi, Rolling Stones, Queen, or any other familiar pop culture reference growing up in our home. This was not something I bragged about at school, but Scott Hahn and Pope John Paul II were the household names that my siblings and I would have recognized even from an early age. My poor boyfriend did not know what he had gotten himself into.

I was incredibly intrigued by the chasm of difference between the beliefs we shared and the ones we didn't. As months went on into our relationship, a plethora of questions were asked and conversations started. I didn't get very far on my own, so I brought my investigation back to my dad who would explain it all to me, and give me references for all the important details. He would also pose questions for me to ask Nate in hopes of getting him to think more deeply about his own understanding of Scripture. I challenged myself to do the same. His heels were dug just as far into the mud as mine.

He was very accepting of my personal beliefs as a whole, but I wasn't so charitable. I just wanted him to convert—which was far from the right attitude for me to have. I'm sure you can see how this relationship was only going to go so far, but I wasn't so willing to arrive at that conclusion voluntarily. He was my first love and this was my first serious relationship. I was too stubborn to take the hard, honest look at our future that was necessary—so, Hurricane Katrina did it for me.

I had just begun my sophomore semester at UNO when Katrina began to threaten our gulf coast. Nate and I had been together for about eleven months and saw each other almost daily, but the impending danger lurking just beyond Louisiana's shores sent us evacuating with our families in different directions. My family traveled west to my aunt's home near Lafayette, which was removed from the worst path of destruction, but still felt the effects of the storm. With no cell service, Nate and I lost touch for a while.

Our city back home was under water, so we remained transplanted for about a month. We were finally able to meet up at LSU in Baton Rouge just to say hello, but it was apparent that things were different between us. Interfaith relationships can certainly work, but our deep personal convictions were polarizing and we were finally feeling its effects.

After we all made it back home, he asked if I would meet him on the levee in Rivertown where there was a pier and some benches (this was a river levee that was never at risk of collapsing from the storm). I had missed him so much that I was just excited to see him and hoped to reconnect any lines that may have been dropped. But *he* had taken our time apart to assess the stability of our relationship appropriately, concluding that we were not called to be together. It initially felt like I was blindsided, but I knew in my heart that he was right. I would later fall apart, but God gave me every grace I needed to accept the news with tact. I sincerely appreciate how delicately Nate handled my heart that night. It was the first and last time we said "I love you."

The next few weeks and months were hard, and for various reasons. I was trying to get cleaned up from heartbreak number one and *still* trying to reconcile the discrepancies in my understanding of the Catholic faith where Nate had challenged me in so many different ways. We ultimately broke up due to our faith differences, but what if I was wrong about Catholicism? With the emotional blow of my first heartache, all kinds of doubt began to creep in. For the first time in my life, I started to seriously question whether or not I was a card carrying member of the Church Christ Himself started.

Finally, it hit me like a ton of bricks that I was only Catholic because it was the faith my parents handed down to me. It had never occurred to me that living out Christianity in light of my Catholic faith was a decision that needed to be made personally––and daily. I now had a responsibility to honestly and unbiasedly assess Scripture and dive deep into prayer to figure out what was true and what diverged from truth at some point in history. I had to make the decision to be Catholic for myself. Thank God, I was ultimately confirmed to be in the right place at a time where I fell even more deeply in love with my rich Catholic faith. It was not without great pain and work, but God had a purpose through it all. You might even say I was "reborn."

Dominic

My older sister, Angela, was about fifteen years old when she experienced her first serious relationship. She was always more mature than me in many ways. I was a young ten years old at the time and was thrilled to have another brother figure to take an interest in, but also to bother when the situation called for shenanigans. Thomas was always very sweet to me and made me feel very special as his girlfriend's little sister. You're not far off if you are interpreting that there may have been a little crush kindling underneath the surface. This is why it was so funny when I started dating his little brother about ten years later.

I stayed involved in my youth group well into college, now serving as a Core Team member in the Life Teen at my local Church parish. Nate had attended Mass and Life Teen with me several times, and even traveled to a Steubenville Youth Conference with our parish. Some time after Nate and I broke up, Dominic became a Life Teen Core Team member with me. Core Team members participated in the planning and carrying out of various activities and events during the "Life Nights" after Sunday mass, for service projects, and yearly retreats under the leadership of the Youth Minister. We also went to UNO together and he ended up joining the Catholic organization that Nate helped me to start on campus. This is how we got to know each other better.

Dominic is very athletic. We bonded over our appreciation for sports and a spirit of fierce competition. Angela and Thomas were not much different when they were together. We even facilitated a fundraising volleyball tournament for our youth group, which was kicked off by a two-on-two match: My sister and I versus Thomas and Dominic, which included a terrifying amount of trash-talking.

We also enjoyed going to movies and watching TV together, which was a relaxing contrast to my prior non-stop relationship which didn't leave much time for fun and brainless activities. We shared several close friends who we bonded with over board games, but these were not your typical game nights. We made Cranium, Taboo, and charades look like gladiator matches. There wasn't a whole lot of depth to our relationship, but I genuinely appreciated the freedom of sharing all the same beliefs and many of the same interests. I had every intention of sticking with it to see where it might go because it wasn't easy to find a good Catholic man who met all three important features of my list. And he introduced me to sushi. Nevertheless, our relationship didn't last very long and I was shocked when he told me why he was ending it.

One evening we ended up in the parking lot of Lafreniere Park. We slowly walked along the white cement ground divided by bright yellow stripes, occasionally balancing on top of the curbs framing each spot. He delicately led into his polite rejection of any potential future together, but I can't remember anything else he said besides "I believe God is calling me to be a priest."

Once my surprise wore off, I, of course, objected to this notion. But he was right. He was so right that you can now find Fr. Dominic at the same parish where we helped to lead Life Teen many years ago as the newest Pastor. I even sometimes find him downstairs at my house playing poker or participating in Fantasy Football drafts with my husband and his friends who all run in the same crowd (Yea, but it's only *kind of* weird).

I didn't see the priesthood *or* the break up coming. So, even though there wasn't a whole lot of grieving to do due to the lack of depth *and* the fact that I was stepping aside for Jesus Himself, I had to embrace my next mourning period as I got cleaned up for the second time.

But at least my sister and I won that volleyball game.

Jake

Jake was the one that wiped the floor with me. I had brushed off the shocker of being dumped for the seminary, was finishing up my last year or so of undergrad, and enjoying life with my people. I had an incredible group of friends who love Jesus and were of like mind and faith practice who I both played and worshipped with. I remain close friends with most of them today.

I had recently turned twenty-one years old and ran into one of my girlfriends at the CCRNO Young Adult Conference. Many refer to Lindsay as the "walking Jukebox" because she has always been a consistent source of entertainment by singing songs of various genres ranging from Gospel to hip hop. Our similar appreciation for rap music was one of the many things that drew us together. During our chat at the conference, she mentioned that she had someone she wanted me to meet. He was "extremely hot," a devout Catholic with a recent conversion, loved sports, "is a little ghetto," and very single—because he was seeking a good Catholic girl (slowly raised hand).

I was intrigued. Lindsay was a "house mom" living at the boys house of *Boys Hope Girls Hope*, "help[ing] academically motivated middle and high school students rise above disadvantaged backgrounds and become successful in college and beyond." My friends and I spent some time hanging out there with the kids and house parents, so she arranged for Jake and I to meet at a game night she organized. I put on my cute jeans and a little makeup and the rest was history. We instantly connected, falling hard and fast.

We were equally fervent in our love and passion for our Catholic faith, enjoyed what I considered to be a surprisingly rich emotional intimacy, had fun whether we were watching TV on the couch, doing homework, or out at a T.I. concert. He would just sit on the phone with me when my cramps felt like they were tearing my insides apart.

It was during this time that the progress I made towards a deeper personal relationship with Christ, originally initiated with Nate, entered into full bloom. Jake was the first person I knew that had truly encountered suffering in his life from when his twin brother died of a brain tumor at only seven years old. It still weighed heavily on him to some extent and I learned a lot from his sincerity and vulnerability as he opened up to me about this. He was not shy about sharing himself without leaving out his pain. He first told me he loved me through a whisper in the adoration chapel. True story! He said, "It's ok if you're not ready to say it, but I am in love with you."

And although I was completely smitten, I *wasn't* ready to say it yet. Remember how seriously I took dating? Remember how I had had my heart broken twice by now and got a real taste for how these things can end? I loved him hard, but was terrified to allow myself to sink deep into this relationship like I so desperately wanted to. Jake was aware of this and was patient with me. He recognized that my heart was guarded and expressed his desire to grow closer by comparing it to rooms in a house, saying, "You've let me into the kitchen and the office, but I want to see the rest of the house." No, he wasn't trying to get into the bedroom––there were struggles, but we actually had a very pure relationship. He simply desired depth. I fought it, but it didn't take long for my heart to break through the walls I had formed around it. I eventually became pretty confident that this was my future spouse.

He agreed.

I was about to graduate from college and he had a solid fulltime job, so the discussion wasn't out of the question. We talked about timing, finances, and careers, and engagement became something that was realistic within the next few years. With all this in the background of our time together, we were happy.

Until one dreadful day came along.

We were studying together in my sister's old bedroom and I could tell that something was bothering him. Although he wasn't ready to open up to me about it, I pressed him for answers. The words that dripped out of his mouth left me stunned. "I feel like God might be calling me to be a priest."

I'm sorry, what? I don't think I heard that correctly. Could you say that again?

He didn't *want* it to be there, but he had been feeling a desire for the priesthood that he could no longer ignore. He was torn right down the middle between this possible calling and his desire to be with me.

I was speechless.

Was he kidding? Could this really be happening **again**?

Isn't there a limit to the amount of times this should happen to a woman? How can I compete with God? *What on earth* did this mean for our relationship?

We entered into a serious discernment about our life together and wrestled with our predicament daily. They don't discuss things like this during homilies at mass. It was a nagging mosquito that robbed our next several months of joy. We needed to be put out of our misery.

By this time, I had become the Youth Minister at another local parish and Jake joined the leadership crew for a Steubenville Trip to Atlanta that I organized and led. If you have ever experienced one of these trips combined with those fruitful bus rides to and from multiple state lines, you know they are special. On our way home, we cozied up in two adjoining seats for a difficult, but intimate moment which called for a decision to be made. We agreed that we needed to take time apart with no contact so he could truly discern God's Will, not unlike the unplanned time that Nate and I were separated post-Katrina. I guess that should've been a warning sign. We settled on three months and it didn't feel rough––it felt impossible.

Still, we were diligent and kept to our plan. Well, he kept to our plan. As the two-month mark approached, I was ready for an update. I needed to hear his voice, so I carved out the worst possible time during a long commute to a morning Physics class to initiate what would become an infamous phone call in my memory. I pulled out of the driveway and tapped his name on my phone. I became more anxious with each ring, which was eventually interrupted by an emotionless "hello."

My heart was ready to burst by the time we finally spoke, yet I found him to be relatively cold and had no idea what to make of it. We chatted for a short time which left me perplexed. I hadn't driven three blocks before he shared with me that he had reached a conclusion to a question I didn't even know he was going to ask. I will never forget the graphite paved intersection, stop sign, and two story hardie-boarded house in my view when I heard his words.

"Mary, I am still discerning whether or not to enter the seminary...but priesthood or not, we are not going to be together."

Time stopped. My ears went deaf and my lips went numb as I was lucky to keep control of my car. I believe it was a handful of angels and the grace of God that allowed me to make it to my class safely. I walked into the school like a zombie and was a waste of a student for the next hour and a half since I heard nothing the teacher said. Fortunately, my class ended in time for me to make noon mass at one of my favorite New Orleans' Churches, St. Anthony of Padua. I had gained enough lucidity to make it to the very last pew. I sat through the entire mass just resting in God's presence with my head in my hands, trying to make sense of the atomic bomb that had just been dropped in my lap without warning.

To say I stumbled through the next several months would be generous. After one meeting post break up, he never contacted me again. There was no closure and I still wonder why he handled the end of our relationship without care. The only conclusion I could come to was that he was an on-fire, baby convert when we met. He was still in a fresh honeymoon-with-Jesus phase that would fade as time passed and the reality of life came pounding. I had been living and growing in the depth of faith I was experiencing at the time and the *on-fire* version of him was the only one I knew. The early highs of a budding relationship had worn off, and it became clear that I was not someone he would choose to love. I parted with an unrecognizable variation of the guy

I thought I'd marry—not unlike the unrecognizable variation of myself that God would begin to clean up after heartbreak number three.

My Catholic faith had already been tested. This break up would begin to challenge my relationship with God. I became bitter because I couldn't grasp why he would allow me to experience such a rich spiritual and emotional connection only to rip it away to keep for Himself. I became bitter because he was now taking a second man from my life to keep for Himself. I became bitter because *how was I supposed to open my heart to another Catholic man,* ever again? I literally felt like God was the "other woman" who stole my boyfriend, yet I was still called to love and serve Him! I wasn't *just* bitter, but absolutely heartbroken. It had been shattered by two men I loved, one on earth and One in heaven.

Time became my best friend. Days turned into months, which helped the shock to wear off and helped me to slowly begin to trust God again. This was my first *real* test of emotional suffering which would have me begging God to make sense of it all. It would take even more time for my heart to internalize the message, but He made it clear to me that this guy was not the one He was calling me to marry. Of course, I couldn't fathom it at the time, but He had someone *much* better in mind.

Miles
Miles is a special person with a heart of gold. I was still a recovering mess when I met him as the newest core team member for the youth group I was still in charge of. He attended Fordham University in New York and came home to Harahan, Louisiana, for the summer to visit family and friends. Football and rugby were two of his passions, which he pursued on teams at West Virginia and Fordham Universities.

I had recently graduated from UNO and was just about to begin the school which would train me to become a Physical Therapist Assistant. My love of sports and desire to help people combined well for this profession. Miles was sweet and fun and we had our love for Jesus, Catholic faith, and athletics in common. He was great with my family, incredibly patient, and a really good listener. We both shared about what we had been through in past relationships. When it came time to talk about Jake, he could tell it was a sore spot.

I discussed the situation minimally at first, but over time, Miles was actually interested to hear about the depth of our relationship and the heartache that followed and appeared to be so profound. He was a good man who wanted to hear my heart and pray for healing, but it was admittedly unusual for it to become such a frequent topic of conversation.

Sometime after Miles and I started dating, I learned through the grapevine that Jake had entered the seminary and I knew this to be a discernment process just like dating was. Eventually, I began to fear that, deep down under my scarred over heart, and despite his blatant rejection of me, there may be some lingering hope that seminary wouldn't stick. I wondered what I would do if I ever got a random text from Jake telling me he had left.

I did eventually get a random text, but it wasn't from Jake. My walking jukebox friend, Lindsay, contacted me to tell me that Jake had officially left the seminary. My stupid brain and heart began to bounce off of each other like a fierce racquetball game. Of course, I began to forget the real reason he ended things as my imagination grew embarrassingly wild. But thankfully, God would overshadow that wonder with reminders of how he ended things *and* how he had become a person I didn't recognize.

I also remembered the striking words that God had impressed so clearly upon my heart promising someone better. The final stage of my healing and metamorphosis (defined by New Oxford American Dictionary as "the process of transformation from an immature form to an adult form in two or more distinct stages") was at bay.

I realized I didn't need Jake, but would have liked some closure. I knew things had changed long before he entered seminary, but the topic had become such a significant part of our relationship and some aspect of its end that I was hoping he would reach out and extend me the courtesy of a text to personally update me. I wasn't looking for a date. I was looking for a more-kind memory of the end of our relationship. So, I did something kind of bold and texted him such, in so many words, to which he responded, "I don't owe you anything."

And he was right––but the *way* he continued to communicate that message to me was not. However, it allowed me to see the parts of him from which God was clearly saving me. I finally felt free.

Don't worry, I haven't forgotten about my dear friend, Miles. That was actually the thing––I eventually realized that Miles had become nothing more than a very dear and selfless friend. He carried me through an entire year of healing I desperately needed, but it was time to say goodbye. And for the first time in my life, I put on my big girl pants and took an honest look at a relationship that wasn't going anywhere. In what I hope was a way that was respectful and gentle on his heart, I ended it.

It was by no means a reflection of the beauty of Miles' heart, but I didn't grieve the end of our relationship. I was sad that I no longer got to spend time with someone I had formed an excellent friendship with, but my heart was not broken. It was *fertile* and perfectly ripened to receive the man God intended for me to spend the rest of my life with.

I'll give you one guess, though, as to where Miles ended up for at least a short time. And yes, I am telling the honest-to-God truth...

The seminary.

Chris

I'm not sure whether I should regard it as a compliment or an insult that I've sent three men into the seminary. Either way, I have considered offering my services to the Archbishop as a part of the vetting program. If the hopeful Seminarian connects with me, they're probably a good fit––at least for a little while.

You better believe I approached my next Catholic boyfriend with caution considering this apparent trend. But thankfully, by the time I met my husband, God had transformed me into a more confident woman who had learned to appreciate that love is a choice with no guarantees and which sometimes hurts. A lot.

You'll learn all you need to know about Chris soon. For now, I just want you to understand that although he is very cute, very athletic, and very in love with Jesus, he is not the type of person I expected to gravitate towards. He doesn't shout his faith from the rooftops like many before him, but is an amazing and incredibly hard-working man who lives it to the core. He has added many traits to my three-criteria-list that I had no idea needed to be there. Dreams of our very own Prince Charmings are often decked out with good looks, talents, and riches, but what really makes a girl feel loved is how well he chooses to enter into suffering with her.

Miles and I had ended up at Chris's house one night for a young adult group prayer meeting that his roommate organized before he and I officially met almost a year later. He didn't initially catch my attention that night, but that house would eventually become my home. He would become my home. He would become the man who frequently sees me at my very worst, at times when I have little or nothing to offer, and in great physical pain, but continues to choose me. Period cramps were a recurrent theme that popped in and out of my life throughout my dating years, but, again, it never once crossed my mind that it may affect my fertility. It was not long after Chris and I started dating that my pain took a turn for the worst, kicking off what would become my next long and winding road of suffering, setbacks, but ultimately great joy.

We all have a certain way that we plan for our life to turn out, but we don't have the same vantage point of the God who passionately loves and desires for us to be incredibly joyful before, and even more so after, all the very messy clean ups that life often requires.

CHAPTER 3

Him

"Let us love, since that is what our hearts were made for."
— Saint Therese of Lisieux

HE HAS A LITTLE BIT of a temper and I can hold a solid grudge. We are sometimes awful at communicating *and* about stealing bed sheets, drive each other crazy on occasion, and only one of us likes country music (it ain't me), but there is no one in the world I would rather suffer and smile with. And boy, have we had plenty of opportunities to suffer together! It's a good thing I learned so much from each previous relationship that led up to him.

Chris has the hard-working heart of a Saint. You know how people describe the heroic love of being able to step in front of a bus to save someone else, but you wonder if you could ever do it if the opportunity ever presented itself? You might get thrown off by his fierce competitiveness and snarky sense of humor, but do not think for one moment that Chris won't be the one to shield a loved one from a ton of oncoming steel.

He wasn't a stranger to suffering either. He had also recovered from the traumatic demise of a serious relationship that ended about the same time Jake wiped the floor with me. Friends had been crucial to helping both of us get through that very difficult time, and it turned out that we had quite a few in common.

We later figured out that we crossed paths multiple times, but had never spoken one word to each other. I ended up running into one of his closest comrades and work buddies, and his wife Ashley, at a Catholic conference at which we were volunteering. Ryan and Chris are cut from the same cloth. They both graduated from UNO with engineering degrees, both work for the same company in the oil and gas field, both love to be on the water in their boats and in their own backyards, and both thrive for creating unique and meaningful projects to serve home and family, both big and small. Their treasured friendship continues to this day.

Ryan had received a call from Chris's mom sometime prior, who didn't know his phone number, so she looked him up in the phone book. (Isn't that cute?) She saw how distraught Chris was from a break up and was desperately hoping Ryan would talk to him and provide some comfort. Ryan didn't know this sensitive side of Chris, but figured that if his mom was determined enough to search the phone book for his digits, it must be serious.

He followed through and over time, this initiated a quest to find Chris a wife! This was ironic because, knowing what a good man Chris is, he always joked that he would be his "insurance policy." If anything should ever happen to Ryan, Ashley should marry Chris. We still laugh about it. Both he and Ashley, like any good friend would, desired for Chris to find the woman that he deserved. Ryan brought this concern to me when I ran into him at the conference.

"Mary, I have this good friend, Chris. Do you know him?"

I honestly couldn't place him from memory alone.

"He's a great guy! I really want to set him up with someone special *because* he's such a good guy. Let me show you some pictures of him."

He looked remotely familiar.

-scrolls through pictures-

"He's an engineer, loves to play sports, 'is a little ghetto' (yea, he really said that), and loves to have fun. He throws lots of parties––look, here are some pictures from a Luau he threw at his house not long ago. It was awesome!"

I couldn't help but wonder if Ryan had *me* in mind to make this love connection. But I had already crashed and burned down that road of being set up and was *not* feeling like going through that again. I also considered that he was coming on a little strong with it all, but I thought it was endearing and I politely engaged.

"So, can you think of anyone we can set him up with? What about your friend Becky? Do you know of anyone else?"

Well, I didn't see that coming! If he *was* trying to make me Chris's future wife, he was being awfully sly about it. Either way, I was relieved when he said he was looking for someone else. I was able to put my guard down because *now I was needed*. And we all like to be needed.

I whipped out my phone and thought of a few prospects. Ryan told me about how Chris's parents had shared with him that they had been praying for Chris to find a "good, Catholic young woman." Most of my friends were taken, but there was one special girl who I thought he might connect with. So yes, believe it or not, I actually tried to set up one of my best friends with my then future husband.

Hey, at least there was no mention of seminary!

It turned out that Chris was actually a pretty hot commodity. He has a sanguine temperament who knows how to bring people together for a good time. He's the first one to mix up a mojito and kick up the party on the dance floor. You could easily find him on the beach, on a cruise, or on any given Sunday in the Superdome cheering on the Saints. He did not need help getting dates––maybe just a little help connecting with the right ones.

Several weeks passed and Chris and Becky never ended up on that date, but I remembered his name and started stalking his Facebook page without the pressure of having to follow through with anything. I started to become *very* intrigued by this man and started texting Ryan's wife, Ashley, to divulge my blossoming interest. I also chatted with Ryan to find out more and give him the green light. I had no idea what that meant, but I was in a good place and ready to move forward whatever that was going to look like.

Not long before I began to open my mind and heart up to the possibility of letting someone new into it, my good old walking jukebox friend was about to be married. It was an exciting time for her and all of our friends actually. We were at that twenty-something age when there's a new wedding at least every month. It becomes a little expensive, but a lot of fun. Ok, it becomes a *lot* expensive and a lot of fun.

This wedding would be different, though, because it would be the first time I would see Jake after his far-from-cordial second rejection of me. I had finally moved on from that saga which had ultimately shaped me into a more confident and sophisticated version of myself. I had no desire to speak to him, but would let my appearance do the talking. And it did. I looked good and took lots of pictures to prove it, which were subsequently posted on Facebook.

Several months later, I found out that I wasn't the only one doing some Facebook stalking. Ironically, Chris was the first to break the ice by commenting on one of those very photos: "Pretty pic!" I was surprised and touched. He had taken notice of me and opened the door for a slow, but certain path to our budding relationship.

We talked over Facebook messenger for a while before exchanging phone numbers. He told me about his three siblings, their spouses, and the ten children (now eleven) that exist between all of them. We texted about Saints football and beach volleyball. He had season tickets and both of us were on teams at our local sand volleyball court, known to locals as "Coconut Beach." We enjoyed some healthy trash-talking, but talking was about all that was happening. It took us several weeks to see each other in person for the first time. His heart was extremely guarded from his previous break up.

Our first date finally came and was notable. He drove to my house after a Sunday Saints game that ran late to pick me up for Mass then bowling. As Mass was ending, I noticed his shirt was on inside out from rushing after the football game. Then he introduced me to his friends as "Megan." *Ha!* You might have thought this date was a disaster, but it was perfectly memorable the way it was. Evidently, I did some random, but cute dance after I bowled a spare, which he still describes as the *thing* that really made me stand out and made him want to get to know me more.

Ryan and Ashley finally admitted that it *was* their intention to bring us together all along, those sly dogs. Well played Ryan, well played. Evidently, Chris had jokingly given Ryan *his* list of ideal criteria in a woman, but I did happen to fit the bill:
1. Athletic/active - check
2. Petite - check
3. "A little ghetto" - check

Awesomely Awful
We grew closer over the next several months, but Chris's heart was not easily willing to move at the same pace as mine. I had good days and bad days when it came to showing him patience and giving him the time he needed to let me in on his own terms. But he was actually invested in me and our future more than I realized.

When we started dating, I had already been roughing it through painful periods for about twelve years. I was a pro. But my pain started to increase significantly as we began to develop a fairly serious relationship. Chris and I had been together for only about seven months when I finally got my endometriosis diagnosis with a side of potential infertility at twenty-four years old. I played that conversation out in my head: "Let's discern marriage. Oh, you have a big family and are eager to have children? By the way, I just found out that I may not be able to have any..." is a great conversation starter for the end of a relationship.

Remember, I was naive when it came to expectations of achieving pregnancy even with a disease that has a reputation for attacking a woman's fertility. I also did not anticipate my pain getting as severe as it did. Just because I wasn't worried about being infertile doesn't mean he shouldn't have been, but he never batted an eye or made me feel as though this new diagnosis was going to be a factor in planning our future together. He continued to choose me for who I was and not for what I was able to give him—or not give him. *That* is love. I would eventually learn how to love my own self in that way.

He romanced me during the next several months in ways that no girl dreams of, but all women yearn for. Chris devoutly cared for me during my first three surgeries and recoveries, and flew with me to Omaha, Nebraska, at two different times for two different procedures as he worked long-distance. It gave him the opportunity to serve me like a superhero and as he stepped up, I fell even more in love with him.

I knew this was my future spouse. He proposed to me on the rooftop of Jax Brewery opposite the St. Louis Cathedral and overlooking the Mississippi River right before my third surgery, which would be my most physically challenging one by far. Everything was beautiful. Two days later, I walked into my pre-op beaming with my new rock weighing down my left hand. His timing revealed that not only did he know what he was getting into, but that he would continue to choose me no matter what. His actions revealed how a real, selfless man responds in stressful situations, and how I deserve to be treated. The quality of a relationship is not determined by how great the highs are, but how we choose to love each other during the challenging lows.

His self-sacrifice was not only evident to me, but to my brother and father who are not easily impressed. They both publicly commented at our rehearsal dinner on his humble and heroic presence throughout what could have been a very dark time. Two days later, we sealed our bond with wedding rings, but the challenges didn't stop. Pain would begin to approach in new forms, we learned that pregnancy would not come easily, and more surgeries would be scheduled. The way Chris continued to step into servanthood during these early trials made me instantly grateful, even though the beginning of our marriage did not turn out as expected.

Only because of *him*, I remember the early years of our marriage to be awesome. I recognized that I had been gifted not only with him, but with a greater and deeper understanding of love and appreciation for the Sacrament. Granted, I am a very lucky woman. But raving about my husband is not the purpose of this chapter. Besides giving some more context, I hope to convey something that I have learned through my witness of his actions. Love is a choice that every single one of us can make daily. No matter what we did or *didn't do* yesterday, or how much we screwed up years before that, love is a choice that we get a new opportunity to make every single morning. It never goes out of style or becomes wasted. It only bears fruit. And I am so grateful that God reserved me to be loved by him. All of this knowledge came in handy as we began to learn about and live through our infertility, which can easily hijack the intimacy right out of a marriage, and especially out of intercourse.

CHAPTER 4

Why Not Birth Control?

"God keeps the entire Universe in order, and still finds time to take a personal interest in you and me."
— *Mother Angelica*

I NEVER IMAGINED THE CHALLENGES I'D experience with my husband early in marriage. I didn't just wake up randomly one morning with killer pains. I didn't know it would become something I would have to plan my life around. I didn't know there was so much I didn't know about my body as a young girl trying to navigate her way into adulthood. In a country that champions women empowerment, self-discovery, **and "choice,"** where were my options? Where was the education about the incredible design of a woman's body I so desperately needed? What about my feminine genius? If the theology of the body illuminates the language of love our bodies are supposed to speak, why was my fertility, and its intimate connection to my health, so often left out of the conversation?

There were many opportunities for conversations to be had in my Catholic schools, youth groups, doctor's offices, and even TV shows that frequently shine a light on important topics. And I truly believe that lack of communication added years of pain to me and stole years of potential fertility from me. Although I do feel failed by some of the faithful on earth, I wholeheartedly appreciate the source of truth that Christ's Church remains and the fruit that is born from Her direction. Pope St. Paul VI, and one man in particular that he has inspired, have become two of my greatest heroes. Still, we have a lot of work to do in our culture and our churches. Let me tell you about how I got here...

The Catholic Church is the only church that continues to stand firm in her denunciation of birth control as a life giving and vow honoring option for spacing children, but that hasn't kept a large number of Catholics from using it. Also, consider that avoiding pregnancy is not the only use for birth control. According to a Guttmacher Institute study[2] (2011), if you know four people experiencing some type of pain or dysfunction associated with menstruation, at least two of them are on birth control.

You don't need to know a whole lot about the drug or a woman's body to be aware of how commonly it is used for a variety of reasons in our culture. If you're slightly more familiar with this scenario, you know that this drug is also peddled to "preserve" fertility until one is ready to try and achieve pregnancy. When you read about all the pain, surgeries, and infertility I have had, you might wonder, "Woman, why have you never considered birth control?!"

Well, I have considered it. You can't make a well-informed decision if you don't understand all of your options. And it is licit to use birth control for medical reasons (as long as sex does not occur during a period of breakthrough ovulation), but that doesn't make it a good, healthy option. In order to fully understand my answer to that question, I need to tell you the stories of a few firsts: my first period, my first couple of doctors, and my very first surgery.

I began experiencing some form of cramps before my first period ever. I learned later that this is not all that unusual for girls with endometriosis. It was an unfamiliar pain I began to have periodically, which I responded to by lying on the couch. When 'Aunt Flow' finally visited at age thirteen, it became obvious what was causing these visits to the sofa.

The pain increased as years passed, but the unspoken cultural rule that pain with periods is normal and should be tolerated as such put a hard stop to any possibility of seeking to understand *why* I was experiencing so much discomfort, and then to subsequently address it at an early age.

As a faithful Catholic, I was familiar with the idea of Natural Family Planning (NFP), but was unaware that there were multiple well-researched options with strong medical components to choose from—one of which has a highly successful medical and surgical application for my women's health problems and even has its roots firmly planted in Catholic soil. (Find support and the information you need on *all* methods at www.fabmbase.org.)

That response of silence to my growing health problem clearly took on many forms and would ultimately allow my undiagnosed disease to progress significantly, attacking my reproductive organs.

I wasn't sexually active, so I didn't have that infamous first pap smear until I was about nineteen years old. Since I was there and my doctor was checking things out anyway, I figured I'd mention that my periods *did* seem to be unusually painful and heavy. I bled through my school skirt one morning in Latin class and over the years, the pain had become harder to tolerate. I hoped this would persuade her to do some investigating––you know, like doctors generally do when you present them with symptoms.

But unfortunately, that's not what gynecologists typically do.

She didn't ask me one question about my cycle or symptoms, nor did she perform or order any further tests. She simply performed the pap smear and asked me, "What kind of birth control do you want?" Oh, that frustrating and dismissive question will ring in my ears for all of eternity! After talking to many women in similar situations, I know now that this is not an atypical scenario.

I wasn't accustomed to taking any kind of medication up to that point. It had taken me a while to even learn how to swallow pills and I knew nothing of this new drug she was offering me. It made me just uncomfortable enough to decline and walk away disappointed with the promise of cyclic pain and shroud of mystery over the inner workings of my menstrual cycle intact.

About five or six years later––and several months after Chris forgot my name on our first date, I was awakened early in the morning with an intensely sharp pain on one of my ovaries. It fluctuated, but I held my breath when it came because the slightest movement provoked whatever was angry inside of me. I tried to get an appointment with the same doctor who had given me my first pap smear, but had to see the nurse practitioner on such short notice.

She didn't appear to take my description of this new pain very seriously since she agreed to do an ultrasound only with the stipulation that she wouldn't add an extra charge if she found something that could be causing the pain. She made me feel like an inconvenience. She was shocked to find that I had an unusual cyst on one of my ovaries and ordered a full ultrasound to be done by a technician on another day. After this second examination, no one got back to me with the results.

Months later, the same pain returned and I found a new doctor at a different hospital who was able to get me in right away. I found her to be much more sympathetic, and even interested in the cause of my discomfort. She immediately sent me down the hall for an ultrasound. The technician reacted to something she was seeing on the screen and called the doctor in.

Diagnosis

On that day, which happened to be my twenty-fourth birthday, Dr. New Gyno threw a fancy six syllable word at me that I had never heard in my life. "Have you ever been told you may have en-do-me-tri-o-sis?

That was a hard no. It had taken twenty-four years for me to be introduced to a disease that is not uncommon, affecting one in ten women. One common symptom of many is glaringly obvious and easy to identify: pain. What only adds to the perplexity of this situation is that it takes, on average, anywhere from seven to twelve years to get a diagnosis. But why? My opinion is that young girls who complain of cycle pain often get brushed aside, or don't mention it all, in an effort to comply with that unspoken rule suggesting that we *just deal with it.*

Whether we are taken seriously or not, mainstream gynecology's immediate solution is usually to prescribe hormonal birth control, which introduces daily synthetic hormones into the woman's system with the intention of shutting the fertile system off by suspending ovulation. This often relieves the woman, or girl, of her symptoms, so she goes on with her life. However, there is no investigation into or treatment of the underlying problem. If symptoms are being caused by endometriosis, research shows that birth control does not prevent the progression of the disease. So, time passes with no diagnosis because few will analyze/address the cause of the symptoms before it becomes a bigger problem. I didn't know any of this at the time, but learned more as years passed and it became more apparent that I was becoming another victim of this machine.

Endometriosis is a disease characterized by cells that resemble the ones that line the uterus (endometrium) implanting on areas outside of the uterus. Lesions can be located anywhere in the pelvic cavity, and less commonly, in other locations of the body and it is progressive, which means that it tends to grow over time. Since endometrial cells become inflamed and shed cyclically during each period, endometriosis causes an additional inflammatory response wherever these lesions are located and can result in pain, scar tissue, and infertility.

This disease can technically only be diagnosed through surgery. But I had a four centimeter blood-filled endometrioma (called a "chocolate cyst") on one of my ovaries that pretty much gave the disease away––not that it was even trying to hide. To give you some perspective, an ovary is normally about the size of an almond, three to five centimeters. Functional cysts on the ovaries are *not* filled with blood, so she knew this wasn't normal and scheduled me for surgery that day. Happy birthday to me.

The One that Made it Worse

I was actually quite relieved to finally get a potential explanation for the pain I had been living with for about twelve years now. And my new doc was a much better fit as she listened to me and assured me that I wasn't crazy. Endometriosis can be very tricky because unless there is an endometrioma like in my case, the only non-surgical evidence of the disease is subjective. This is another reason why many girls and women feel awkward (crazy, really) for insisting that something isn't right. After she walked me back down the hallway into the treatment room, she discussed surgery and the next order of business with me: birth control.

"Oh man," I thought. "Here we go with the birth control again." But this time was different. Dr. New Gyno actually communicated a caring attitude towards me. She had compassion and desired for me to be free of pain with the ability to achieve pregnancy intact for whenever that option would become available. She insisted that I begin taking the drug immediately and continue even after surgery in an effort to keep symptoms at bay and "preserve" my fertility. The latter was a theory which I later discovered to be without foundation. I shared my hesitancy with her and maintained that I would think about it, so she gave me some free samples to take home as I did some research.

I learned that although it does often eliminate painful symptoms, that is not always the case––and it often adds a wide variety of other unwanted symptoms. It decreases a woman's risk of some cancers, but increases the risk for breast cancer, cervical cancer, and liver cancer. It is considered a Class 1 carcinogen by the World Health Organization[3] and increases a woman's risk of developing a blood clot, which could be deadly.

It doesn't address the underlying problem causing the symptoms nor does it "regulate" the cycle. It just attempts to shut the system down, and it is successful most of the time. The bleed that occurs somewhat regularly when a woman is taking these synthetic hormones is *not* any form of a period, which involves the healthy sloughing off and replacement of the lining cells of the uterus. It is a bleed that results from synthetic hormonal withdrawal alone, which occurs after taking the placebo pill. It is nothing more than a chemical effect.

That isn't even the worst of it. What would I do when I got married and started having sex? It turns out that the role of hormonal birth control is to end the life of a newly conceived baby when breakthrough ovulation occurs (ranging from 1.7%-28.6% per cycle with standard birth control pills and 33%-65% with progestin-only contraceptives[4]) and conception follows, but before the woman would even know she's pregnant. That's because the pill is designed to thin out what should be a thick, nutritious lining of the uterus as another "line of defense" against implantation—just in case it misses the mark of preventing ovulation and sperm transport, and conception occurs.

And wait a minute—isn't surgery supposed to work? Why should I have to have surgery and take the pill? I could not bring myself to put this foreign substance into my body. I was counting on this surgery to appropriately address this disease once and for all. I *needed* it to be successful, after all, I had been educated on no alternatives.

My mom accompanied me to my pre-op where we were educated on the procedure, possibilities, and expected outcomes. I told her that I had decided against using birth control. Dr. Gyno explained that the surgery should relieve my symptoms and there was not enough confetti in the world to supply the party I'd be throwing after that happened. She continued to explain, however, that there could be microscopic endometriosis that she couldn't see, in which case she couldn't remove it, and it could get worse (I guess that's why she wanted me on birth control?). Then she put a sheet of paper in front of me and handed me a pen as she described her intention to do everything she could to keep my reproductive organs intact, but if she would determine that the disease and scar tissue are too severe, she wanted my permission to remove one or both ovaries, tubes, and/or my entire uterus. Just like that. While I was unconscious on an operating table.

And *just like that*, I put my fertility in her hands. At the time, I didn't know any better. We were kind of "happily" (because finally there were answers and hope for relief) blindsided with a diagnosis and surgery, and humans tend to trust doctors blindly. There was a lot of information being given all at once and everything was happening very quickly. We had no choice but to trust the only doctor we knew who'd pay any attention to the dysfunction in my body. I signed my name on the dotted line having no idea how close I was cutting it.

I woke up from the one and half hour surgery with my first three stripes, which would eventually turn into permanent scars, external evidence of deep cuts into my belly and what would eventually become, metaphorically, deep cuts into my heart. I was groggy and nauseous from the anesthesia, but I did prefer that over the bowel prep that made for a miserable evening prior. Dr. Gyno came to visit me in my recovery room and explained that all my organs were accounted for (thank God). She mentioned that she considered removing an ovary, but ultimately decided against it. Bring on the confetti! I went home that day, eager to leave those days of bad cramps behind me.

But weeks passed and my experience of pain remained the same.

I tried desperately to find any ounce of relief during Flow's visit. I considered that maybe I needed to give it some more time, but her second and third visit after surgery brought just as much pain. After only three short months post-op, I was back in my doctor's office for another ultrasound which revealed that a new six centimeter endometrioma had replaced the one she removed and was now accompanied by an additional smaller one. Surgery number two was scheduled before I could even acknowledge my half birthday. Dr. New Gyno insisted that she planned to be even more aggressive this time, which didn't look good for my reproductive organs. And now, she was *strongly urging* me to take birth control.

Chew on This
Well this got real—real fast. Even my doctor was surprised. When the doctor starts to panic, you know something isn't right. So let me give you something real thick and juicy to chew on.

It is very unusual for girls in my situation to decline birth control. In a large majority of the cases, and especially on the higher dosage of the pill she was recommending for me, pain goes away or is at least drastically reduced. But according to the Journal of Endometriosis and Pelvic Pain Disorders[5], "Postoperative hormonal suppression helps reduce pain symptoms and recurrence of endometriomas, but it does not seem to prevent disease recurrence or progression of peritoneal endometriosis, and has not been shown to improve future fertility.

Postoperative suppression until pregnancy is based on expert opinion only..."

So, maybe the endometrioma recurrence wouldn't have been so dramatic, but would I have been aware that the disease was still rampant if I had been on birth control and wasn't feeling the symptoms? To what extent might the disease have progressed had I not been alerted to the pain until I got off of birth control years later to have a baby? How much less severe would the disease have become had I been actually diagnosed and treated by sixteen years old? eighteen years old? In less than twelve years??

This is the situation countless young girls are in because most are completely unaware of how birth control works, that they have other options, and the importance of understanding the menstrual cycle and its connection to overall health.

It was even before I learned that no improvements had been made after surgery that I discovered the Creighton Model Charting System (CRMS) and began charting. I consider this to be a miniature miracle because I knew little of the method and had no reason to believe I needed additional care yet. The Creighton Model is a method of Natural Family Planning (NFP), or what I prefer to refer to as *Fertility Awareness*, which teaches a woman/couple how to chart her cycles in detail, allowing her to monitor fertility and maintain her own gynecological health. Can I get an amen?

By the time I was awaiting my second operative date, I discovered NaProTechnology. The specific kind of charting I just mentioned is the foundation of "NaPro," giving the associated NaProTechnology medical consultants and surgeons insight into what is going on inside of the woman's body and direction for actual treatment. It's kind of a big deal.

One night when Chris and I were leaving Coconut Beach where we played on a sand volleyball team together, my dad called me and told me to turn on a Catholic radio station to hear Dr. Thomas Hilgers, the creator of this women's health science, discussing *his* approach to women's healthcare. When he said that he never prescribes birth control, I couldn't believe my ears. Not only does he not prescribe it, but I learned later that all potential NaProTechnology physicians have to sign a form promising that they won't prescribe it either to even attend his training.

I was dumbfounded and incredibly intrigued to hear more because, as far as I knew, it was unprecedented for an OB/GYN to *never* (relatively speaking) prescribe this drug. But, according to Hilgers, who practices in Omaha, Nebraska, there was never a good reason to shut the woman's fertile system down. That would simply put a bandaid on the problem. He sought to *fix* the problem.

Which actually made a lot of sense. Even more than that, he described an approach that served the *whole* woman. Her fertility is an integral part of her whole person, not a separate and distinct aspect to be turned on and off. He spoke of women with such a profound respect and appreciation that I hadn't experienced from most people, much less a male *OB/GYN*. It was this point of view that inspired the creation of this kind of medical practice.

NaProTechnology certified surgeons are not the only ones who are able to offer high quality treatment. Physicians like Dr. Patrick Yeung and Dr. Nicholas Kongoasa are passionate about restoring the health of women dealing with endometriosis, and this list is growing.

Both my present doctor (whom I respected) and this guy I heard on the radio said they would perform the same surgery on paper, yet I perceived there to actually be something very unique about the NaProTechnology way of doing things. That night, I made a decision to pursue my next surgery at the Pope Paul VI Institute in Nebraska, which Dr. Thomas Hilgers developed with his wife and the rest of his team. He had been deeply moved by the call in *Humanae Vitae* to men of science to find more options for women. I meant no disrespect to Dr. Gyno, but my fertility was too important to put in the hands of someone who may not fully understand and appreciate it, despite her best intentions.

I kept my local surgery scheduled until I could confirm the details. The Institute had a process for long-distance patients to send at least two cycles of charting and any applicable post-operative reports. Dr. Hilgers would review and respond several weeks later with the green light on the morning of my second pre-op locally, which I attended only to cancel my surgery.

He didn't *just* respond with an approval to head there for treatment though. I received a letter with a detailed evaluation of the two and a half cycles of charting I had mailed him:

"In reviewing the Creighton Model chart, the following observations are made. It reveals intermediate-limited mucus cycles and tail-end brown bleeding. These findings are often associated with hormonal dysfunction, ovulation defects, endometriosis, chronic-low grade endometrial infection, chronic inflammation of the cervix, pelvic adhesions and/or blockage of the fallopian tubes.

I would like to make the following recommendations. You should have a thorough hormone evaluation of your menstrual cycle (without meds), thyroid system dysfunction panel, and a diagnostic laparoscopy, hysteroscopy, and selective hysterosalpingogram with endometrial cultures. I do realize that you have had a laparoscopy in the past; however, the endometriosis was treated in such a way that it has a high recurrence rate and scar tissue formation. I would not recommend you undergo another surgery locally. It is imperative that a gynecologic surgeon use meticulous antiadhesion techniques in order to preserve your fertility. I am very concerned about the "more aggressive" plan for surgery. To me, this indicates removal of the ovary and possible fallopian tube. This would be detrimental to your fertility."

He had never met my doctor, but he had her figured out because he, too, was a product of medical school, which focuses on hormonal birth control as the foundation of treatment. The difference with Hilgers was that he recognizes the disservice that birth control generally does to women and believes that we deserve more. The foundation of NaProTechnology is not birth control, but the information gathered from the woman's body via the charting system. It was so interesting to see *his* plan for preserving fertility–hands-on, surgical and anti-adhesion techniques and researched protocols offering additional natural hormonal support, versus *hers*–birth control.

Without ever having met this man, and from eight hundred thirty miles away, he was able to interpret the language of my body which had been providing this valuable information all along. I just had to find the right person to teach me how to write it down, and then interpret it for me.

After I received his letter, it really made me wonder about how my health and womanhood had been handled for the last decade. God has created my body beautifully! He has designed it to communicate with me daily whether or not I'm paying attention, yet he has equipped me with the ability to gather that information. He has gifted scientific minds with the ability to use that knowledge gained to promote actual healing! This is how the body of Christ is intended to work together. My body was using pain, among other things, to communicate to me that something was wrong early in my teenage years. I didn't know that I should visit my doctor earlier with a symptom like this even though I wasn't sexually active.

By the time I saw my doctor, she brushed off the pain just like the nurse practitioner did several years later. Birth control, a drug that doesn't treat endometriosis, was my only option for treatment. I finally started to get some answers by the time I turned twenty-four years old, giving the disease roughly eleven years to wreak its havoc.

Had I been better educated and empowered by my doctors, schooling, my church, and/or my culture, learning how to read my body and understand what is normal and what is not, and been given access to a doctor like Hilgers early in my teen years when it would've been most appropriate, how much more minimal would the damage have become? How much less pain would I have experienced? How many fewer days of school or work would I have missed? Would I be able to have children?

I will never know the answers to these questions. But I can help empower future generations to avoid having to ask them in the first place.

I took my first plane ride ever to Omaha, Nebraska, with my parents and my boyfriend, Chris, for my second surgery, performed by a colleague of Dr. Hilgers whom he personally trained. It was January, so it was also the first time I experienced real snow, which was pretty cool. What was really beautiful about my even newer gynecologist was that I was never asked to sign away my permission to remove any organ because that wouldn't even be an option in this circumstance. She would take as long as necessary to address this disease, regardless of how complicated it may be.

About seven months after my first surgery *and* after the now six and a half hour operation, I learned that one of the endometriomas had grown to ten centimeters, which in combination with the ovary it was sitting on, resembled a "large orange, or small cantaloupe," according to my post-operative report. I was told that the disease was so extensive, appearing on my appendix, bladder, pelvis, uterus, fallopian tubes, both ovaries, utero-ovarian ligament, multiple areas of my bowel, and in addition to identifying scar tissue, that my Napro doctor was confident that Dr. Gyno would've removed every reproductive organ, had I not canceled surgery at my pre-op.

I had just barely escaped a fate that would have rocked me to my core with little to no notice. I sat in absolute awe as I realized how God had mercifully spared me from awakening from anesthesia to quite possibly being told that any hopes of bearing children had been ripped from beneath me before I could even say "I do." I still remember that moment with gratitude.

Chris and I tied the knot almost exactly one year later on January twelfth. We actually moved our wedding up a few months in hopes of taking advantage of every opportunity we might have to conceive a child after receiving the new information of the rare form of aggressive endometriosis I was "lucky" enough to possess. I was hopeful at first, but with all the damage already caused by such a late diagnosis and ineffective first surgery, what could I really expect?

Months and years passed with no baby. Could this really be happening? I knew they said infertility was a side effect, but does this disease know I'm Catholic?! Does it know how desperately we desire children? Surely I was meant to contribute more to my family and the world than the inability to conceive a child? Obviously, I had other important purposes, but this really threw a wrench into my genius plans. Most of us don't *hope* to have children, but expect it. It's a concrete and specific purpose that pretty much comes pre-written on our life "to do" lists.

Hope was slipping away. The feelings facilitated by each passing infertile month continued to take chunks out of my heart, and my self-worth. I felt the gaping hole inside of a womb that I believed should have been housing a baby. What did this say about me as a woman? What did this say about my purpose as such; as a wife? More feelings of doubt began to stretch a hole that had already expanded too much as my worst day ever approached. It was no surprise that day sent me over the edge.

Part of the problem was that I was so consumed with my feelings. But *"Feeling"* is a tricky, overused word, isn't it? How many times do we confuse it with the definition of "thought" and allow a lie to take root? There's an important distinction to be made here! Thankfully, God is patient as we figure these things out because words–and how we use them towards ourselves, in prayer, and to others–matters. Learning how to distinguish between these messages I am sending has given me some priceless insight.

CHAPTER 5

Don't Smite Pontius Pilate!

"Trust in God's Providence, interfering – as it always does – for our own good."
— *Saint Mary Mackillop*

I HAD CERTAINLY BEEN REJECTED IN the past, from the first volleyball team I tried out for, certain friendships, a boyfriend, the first Physical Therapist Assistant jobs I applied for, and now it seemed like my application for biological motherhood would be denied.

We experience rejection from an array of sources and to varying degrees of intensity on a weekly, and sometimes daily, basis. The first acquisitions editor who rejected my book proposal was incredibly kind and very constructive. But I still wanted to go cry in a corner and give up because I decided I wasn't good enough. Often little lies about who we are and how God created us begin to creep in, sewing doubt and stealing our joy. Hearing lies in and of themselves doesn't necessarily cause damage––but believing them does. When the lie takes root, it can set off a chain reaction of destructive side effects. It takes time, patience, and openness to learn how to respond in a healthy way. But a very good first step *is* to actually respond at all.

If you didn't catch it in the Intro, Chris and I were chosen to be the adoptive parents of a little girl who has been the most perfect fit for our family. Although not a "cure" for infertility, her presence has certainly filled a void in our hearts. Of course, there is a spectrum of the joys of parenting. Occasionally when our little three-year-old gets upset about really important things like not being able to put her hand in the hot oven or me saying the word "great" when she asked me not to, her fit includes screaming and/or hitting. We try to teach her that it *is* important to express our feelings, but in a way that is respectful. It is ok for her to be angry even if mommy and daddy don't understand why or think there is a good reason to be because her feelings matter.

Most parents *want* their children to be forthcoming with their thoughts, desires, and feelings so they can be more useful to them. It gives everyone an opportunity to talk about differences, clarify all new information, and provide comfort and encouragement when needed.

Bella doesn't know that touching a four hundred degree oven will severely burn her hand and instantly make her regret being born—that's why she has parents. Adults typically know better than children do because we have the privilege of seeing a bigger picture. A loving parent will meet the child where he or she is and teach them about life and love. The more trust the child has in their parents, the more the parent can serve them.

They typically understand the frustration of a child who simply cannot wrap their heads around certain concepts. If we can even sort-of appreciate this approach to little humans, how much more perfectly can we expect our Heavenly Father to treat us when we are frustrated? There is no parent more loving and empathetic than our God and there was no child more confused than me.

Chris and I did everything "right "--saved sex for marriage, went to weekly mass, received the other Sacraments, had a desire to do good, etc. It initially made zero sense that pregnancy would not flow as a natural extension of these good works, as if getting the things I want should be the result of my ability to follow the Commandments. *Ha!* It's hard to be reminded that that's not how Christianity works. I would have acknowledged my understanding of Christian values with my words, but I still felt bitter, meeting with a long list of hopelessness frequently over the years: Infertility has made me feel worthless, forgotten/ignored by God, rejected, broken, like I had done something wrong or wasn't good enough, like a bad Catholic, doubting my purpose, believing I was less of a woman—and the list goes on. Does any of this sound familiar?

Guilt became a bully that would pick on me for having these responses to my suffering, but this did not make me *bad*. There is nothing wrong with feeling however we feel in response to any bitter disappointment or ruptured expectation. On the contrary, it is how God created us. I was really comforted to learn in marriage prep that we can't control our feelings—only our actions. No one can tell you that your feelings are wrong.

Read that again. Your feelings are real no matter what they are, so feel them. Then take a break and feel them some more. Allow yourself to feel sad. Disappointed. Confused. Angry. Approach your feelings with curiosity. They are valid no matter what they are.

Thoughts Vs. Feelings

The more mind-blowing nugget of wisdom that marriage prep taught us was the difference between a *thought* and a *feeling*. Our own marriage prep mentors, Lloyd and Jan Tate, literally wrote the manual on *In Home Marriage*

Preparation and they remain good friends of ours today. I have pulled out a paragraph from their training materials to share with you, with their permission:

"Feelings are your interior responses to things. They are spontaneous and usually unconscious. Some such responses are anger, joy, sadness, and frustration. Thoughts, on the other hand, are conscious and somewhat judgmental. People often confuse thoughts or opinions with feelings. Whenever you use the expression 'I feel that...' you are usually expressing a thought and not a feeling. Feelings can usually be expressed in a single word."

So we can *think/believe* that we will never be happy without a pregnancy, or anything else that is important to us, and *think* that joy will never return, and *think* that God has forgotten about and abandoned us, but it does **not** mean that it is true. What facilitates internal conflict is when we begin to *believe* our thoughts, regardless of how little truth there is to them. Our feelings, on the other hand, are real. We *feel* disappointed, betrayed, rejected, sad, lonely, etc. or all of the above. Our thoughts typically precede, or inform, our feelings.

Mr. Lloyd would always say: "Feelings aren't always rational, but they are genuine."

I had all the thoughts and all the feelings and all the fits. Sometimes my fits included screaming and hitting things because I didn't know how to process it or where to put it. It was easier to throw a tantrum than to dig up the root of my pain to confront the source face to face. Because what if I *am* wrong? What if I *am* missing something? What if He *really does* know better? What if He sees more potential in me than I would have *dared* dream about? What if He is *not* calling me to give birth to a child? What if He is?

It was hard to ask those questions honestly, not just because I was afraid to get the answers, but because I didn't necessarily feel like I had permission to have those thoughts in the first place.

At least in the Catholic culture I grew up in, I didn't experience a lot of vulnerability and authenticity about daily and lifetime struggles. I don't remember the experience of priests or others in church acknowledging that living the Christian lifestyle God calls us to is **really hard** and many of us fail frequently. Sometimes we doubt and have hard questions. The beauty of this Christian lifestyle, however, includes using the grace of God to get back up and try again, and repeating that process over and over again. The message I received, whether intentional or not, was a life that consisted mostly of rainbows and butterflies for "good Catholics."

But Christ was not just rainbows and butterflies. Although *He* did not fail, He *did* get angry, He *did* suffer and experience great pain, He *did* know great joy, He *did* deliver truth with honesty, but also with love and sincerity. He didn't get to the Resurrection by skipping over Good Friday. He challenged men and women to look within themselves and work hard to reach their greatest potential and to serve one another. He does not call us to be perfect––just to be obedient, and just to keep trying.

The dam holding my feelings back crumbled with that false positive because I hadn't been honest with myself or God for so long, nor had I been directing my efforts towards the right goal. My blood was bubbling with anger and blame, but at least I had no choice but to finally go to the Source of all love and truth.

To My Past Self...
Looking back, I recognize the plethora of lies that I believed which were largely responsible for the enduring and intense blows infertility brought. There is so much I wish I had known! It was only as God revealed the truth to me over time, and as I stepped into my suffering, that I was able to experience healing depths that continue to go deeper. If I could go back, I would have a thing or two to say to myself...

"If you want to know joy again, acknowledge your feelings *and* the thoughts that facilitate them. Be honest about them to yourself and your Creator—*even when you believe He is responsible.* When we go to Him authentically, we remove some of that burden from ourselves and make room for the truth.

Take all the time you need. Be patient with and kind to yourself. Allow hope back in slowly, but surely. *Pain doesn't have to be absent in order to know healing.* Come to God just as you are. He desires all of you—both the polished and the unpolished! And finally, prepare room within yourself for *His* thoughts, ideas, and plans..."

That last one is tough because it doesn't always *feel* this way, but God is incapable of creating a plan for our lives that isn't perfectly suited for us. We are the ones that are often stumbling to get back on track. Although my feelings were real, they were reflections of thoughts and beliefs that were *not true*. It was too much for me to believe that God actually had bigger and better knowledge about me than I had for myself.

Now back to that pep talk. Please imagine Morgan Freeman as your narrator for these next two parts...

"The truth *is* that you are of great and immeasurable value. Nothing about you is worthless. You are far from forgotten and ignored. You're only waiting for your greater purpose and probably already living it. You are unique and needed in this world *exactly as you are.*

You did nothing wrong to deserve "this." People who achieve and maintain their goals, pregnancy included, didn't do anything morally "right" to deserve "that." Being good enough was never in question. Each day brings new choices and new chances *whether we are successful or not.*

The ability to bear a child and give birth is important and beautiful, but it is a very small aspect of being a woman—even a mother! We nurture, counsel, advise, educate, love, discipline, show compassion and tenderness, listen, serve, laugh, create, and much more and *to* many more than just our own little humans...and for far more than nine months. We are valuable not only to our families, but to our friends and communities who count on *all* of our gifts––not just the ones we give first and last names to. And anything contrary to what I have just told you is the lie."

-End pep talk-

It is hard to see how treasured we truly are––most of us have been unnecessarily beating ourselves up for a while now. But you can accept the wonderful truth about yourself with time. So, you're afraid of failing? Me too! That's okay. There is no limit to your opportunities to choose love for yourself, for God, for others. Choosing to be patient with myself and God, and learning to be still, was the best gift I learned to give myself. We have all heard that He knows our needs more intimately than we do, but the only person who hasn't struggled to internalize that fact is our Blessed Mother. Rome wasn't built in a day, but it was eventually built! There is always hope. And don't let that little jerk (Satan) tell you anything differently.

I knew that God had the ability to bless Chris and I with a healthy pregnancy at any given moment, which is why I was getting so hurt by his apparent monthly decision to keep us waiting. But then I remembered that I am the same person who reads that part of the Gospel when Pontius Pilate convicts Jesus every Good Friday and *still* internally screams "God, just come down and smite Pilate already!!!" at the pages in hopes that Christ will escape His torture.

But He doesn't, nor do we really want Him to, because we know what happens at the end of the story. He doesn't smite Pilate–not because He isn't insanely in love with His cherished Son–but because the Resurrection and all the incredible beauty that follows requires the endurance of the cross.

CHAPTER 6

My New Best Friend

"We are to love God for Himself, because of a twofold reason; nothing is more reasonable, nothing more profitable."
— Saint Bernard of Clairvaux

SO, HOW MANY TIMES HAVE you heard the line about "God's perfect plan?" Are you sick of it yet? Have those words graced your ears during a homily or as they flow beautifully out of a speaker's mouth? How about on paper? I don't personally have enough fingers to hold up. I know I've probably said it a hundred times and it sounds great, but it also sounds cliche. Everybody *knows* God has this wonderful plan for our lives, but more often than not, it feels like we're squinting through a microscope to find even the tiniest pieces of it. That's why that false positive pregnancy test was so hard. Not only could I not get pregnant, but I couldn't get the reassurance of an accurate test window and a little comfort from up above? Boy, please.

But take a moment to prepare yourself for the next stroke of wisdom I'm about to throw your way: you don't actually need to *know* what the plans are to come to be at peace with them. Don't get me wrong–having a roadmap would be splendid, but ultimately, it's how we approach the journey itself that's most important. All I need to know is that God loves me fiercely despite what the lies are telling me. I had to resolve to continue to choose God even as it felt like He was consistently ignoring me. Moving forward was a painful act of the will not unlike physically placing one foot in front of the other when learning how to walk again after breaking a leg. You don't always feel the progress, but you have to keep going. You've got to put in the work, especially when it's really hard.

On top of the infertility I had been dealing with for years, God was still withholding consolation from me after that painful experience on my "worst day ever." But on the following day as I sat on my living room sofa contemplating life and searching for direction in an abyss of loneliness, God dropped some golden bread crumbs for me. As I scrolled through my phone, I stumbled upon some quotes by a woman who was about to become my new favorite saint: the one and only Teresa of Avila (Insert heart emoji here).

"There are more tears shed over answered prayers than over unanswered prayers." (Interior Castle by St. Teresa of Avila*)*
I'm not even completely sure what this is supposed to mean, but it certainly puts a different perspective on prayer and on God's plans for my life. I love how it makes me think.

"In light of heaven, the worst suffering on earth will be seen to be no more serious than one night in an inconvenient hotel."
What a silly, but completely applicable analogy. Her comparison is unusual, but meaningful, and it really puts suffering into perspective.

"I do not fear Satan half as much as I fear those who do fear him." (Interior Castle by St. Teresa of Avila*)*
Here is another series of strange, but useful words. The way she thinks both perplexes and teaches me. It's also starting to make me laugh.

"To reach something good it is very useful to have gone astray, and thus acquire experience." (Interior Castle by St. Teresa of Avila*)*
Yes. Yes. Yes. With a strict background, you tend to either run the other way or do the right thing out of fear or obligation and not out of love. This thought comforts me and reaffirms that God makes use of all of our suffering; our mistakes–even the suffering that is caused by ourselves!

"I don't know what heavy penance I would not have gladly undertaken rather than practice prayer." (Interior Castle by St. Teresa of Avila*)*
Another excellent example of raw *honesty* from this holy woman! Sometimes we don't like to pray. It is just the vulnerable truth, which is not always easy to find in Catholic circles. This statement gave my heart permission to feel human.

"May God protect me from gloomy saints."
Ha! This one made me laugh out loud. What kind of Saint says these things? Um, one that I wanna be best friends with.

And my favorite:
"[Lord,] If this is how you treat your friends, no wonder why you have so many enemies."
I'm pretty sure we all have that last thought at least every other Tuesday, but we aren't saying it out loud. I cannot get enough of her honesty!

As I read through St. Teresa's quotes, I not only felt that she had captured my longings and emotions, but that I could really relate to her *personality* and admire her incredible honesty! I had never heard a Saint talk like this. She felt so refreshingly authentic to me! This was an exhilarating splash of water over my sizzling emotions. Hope began to *very* slowly creep up over the horizon.

A National Catholic Register article[6] describes Avila like this: "[her] descriptions of contemplative prayer and its effect upon the soul are unparalleled. She writes with joyous abandon and humorous, self-deprecating humility, and her writings are accessible to all."

Her words were like a hug. She was my own little sassy, sarcastic saint who had me laughing with a childish grin, while crying & rejoicing simultaneously. She is even a Patroness of those who suffer physical pain. We had an instant connection and I recognized that God had led me to the most perfect heavenly friend who would walk me through my darkest days and help me to continue to choose Him when I wasn't sure what that looked like.

Dark Night
My new pal had gotten my attention and piqued my interest. I thought it was weird that a loving Father would allow me to experience such emotional pain and emptiness, so I wanted to know more. God has what seems to the naked eye to be an unusual way of drawing us closer to him. I soon confided in Casey, a dear friend of mine who was genuinely concerned about my heart and more familiar with theology than I was. It was hard to be close with friends who were fertile at that time, but her sincerity and wisdom were comforting. I explained everything from the darkness of my worst day ever to my new favorite Saint

who was holding my hand as I walked through it. I was surprised to hear that she knew exactly what I was describing.

That was the first day I learned of "the dark night of the soul" as described by St. John of the Cross and, of course, lived out by my new 16th century friend. Casey thought I was experiencing my own miniature "dark night."

In my opinion, Emily Stimpson Chapman describes this "dark night" well in an article published by *Our Sunday Visitor*:

"Every fallen human being has disordered desires and attachments. We love what we shouldn't love, or we love what we should but in the wrong way. We seek our own comfort, our own pleasure, our own will. We value what we want more than we value what God wants. We do wrong, even if only in our hearts.

But we can't do wrong and stand before God. We can't even want to do wrong and stand before God. A prerequisite for seeing God face to face is that every attachment to sin, both in our lives and in our hearts, must be broken. If we want to become saints, we have to desire only God's will. And we have to desire God's will not out of fear of hell, but rather out of love for heaven, out of love for God. Some of that breaking we do, as we learn to avoid vice and pursue virtue. But some of that breaking only God can do. The dark night of the soul is, in part, how he does that. By seemingly withdrawing all spiritual consolations—all the little comforts and supports that typically come from pursuing a relationship with him—and allowing an almost crushing sense of abandonment to descend upon us, he purifies our desires and prepares us for heaven."

Yup, sounds about right! It may seem counterintuitive for a loving God to allow such an awful experience for the sake of greater unity, but it actually makes sense when you consider that love is not a feeling, but a choice—kind of like that time He willingly suffered an agonizing death for us even though He did nothing wrong.

It initially sounds cruel, but with deeper reflection, you can see that God is removing the noise so we can be drawn even closer to Him. He allows only the "sense of abandonment," but **not** abandonment itself. Although I'm sure it is a bit more complicated than described here, and maybe even impossible to fully understand on this side of heaven, my understanding of it is that God desires for us to choose Him despite the complete absence of understanding Him and His will, his comforting presence, and even the most basic luxuries of temporal life. He wants us to choose Him for who He is and not for what He can do for us.

Teresa of Avila was a Carmelite Saint who lived in the 16th Century and persevered through a period of interior darkness that lasted twenty years! This experience was the source of pain calling her to cry out her famous quote about how God treats His friends. But she has quite the collection of incredibly profound quotes which capture the spirit of perseverance and hope through suffering:

"Let nothing perturb you, nothing frighten you. All things pass. God does not change. Patience changes everything."

"Pain is never permanent."

"May today there be peace within.
May you trust God that you are exactly where you are meant to be.

May you not forget the infinite possibilities that are born of faith.
May you use those gifts that you have received, and pass on the love that has been given to you.
May you be content knowing you are a child of God.

Let this presence settle into your bones, and allow your soul the freedom to sing, dance, praise and love.
It is there for each and every one of us."

"You pay God a compliment by asking great things of Him."

"Christ has no body now, but yours. No hands, no feet on earth, but yours. Yours are the eyes through which Christ looks compassion into the world. Yours are the feet with which Christ walks to do good. Yours are the hands with which Christ blesses the world."

These words spoke directly into a heart buried under a weight of feeling forgotten, ignored, and passed over by God. Those feelings couldn't have been farther from the truth because, like every other human, God created me with rich purpose.

Those descriptions of our function as children of God do not exclude women who can't bear children. They exclude no one. I would eventually find a place of acceptance where I would no longer need the answers to all of my questions: Why did it feel like I was the only person not pregnant? Nearly everyone around me was achieving pregnancy so easily! Had I done something wrong? Was I a bad Catholic? Was I being punished? Why am I broken? Were they better than me? That'll be four "no's" for five hundred, Alex. Over the years, Avila has helped to restore me in ways I cannot fully explain.

With incredible patience, God slowly revealed to me that my inability to get pregnant was *allowed* on *purpose*. I was not forgotten, but treasured like everyone else—uniquely reserved to become the person and woman God created me to be and contribute to the world, my family, *and the church*, in a precise way that only I can.

I would not have become the person I am today without my particular cross of infertility. He doesn't desire that we suffer. But along with sin, suffering crept into the world like a sneaky, uninvited house guest. So God allows us to make use of it. It actually brought me great comfort to understand that as hard as it was, I was exactly where I needed to be—*on purpose*, and with *great purpose*.

With this new understanding of life that I am still unpacking, I began to feel less and less despair.

More Colors, Please
I had unknowingly made my own life expectations identical to the roles my mother fulfilled––which she did beautifully, but that doesn't mean they are mine to step into. These roles were congruent with what is often subtly and not-so-subtly passed along as goals for "good Catholic women"—whether it be by clergy, church workers/volunteers, or other good Catholic women. But what was *Mary Bruno* actually made for? And does it have to be limited to just one to three things?

Don't get me wrong––having multiple children, being a stay-at-home mom, homeschooling, and other similar variations are beautiful and needed vocations! But the very fact that infertility exists tells us that there are many different important ways to be fruitful. If every family and their gifts looked the same, the world would be a boring and bland coloring book starving for new and unusual colors. And there would be a diverse group of people thirsting to be ministered to.

God has blessed us with this incredibly colorful world with as many different varieties and appearances of people and their associated gifts as there are pigments of the rainbow. The world needs us each to fully embrace the individual our Father has created us to be and dust off all the gifts and talents He has planted within our very bones to share and give life to those around us. We pay God a great compliment when we do! This is what it means to be truly life-giving; to be fertile.

Among many other wise lessons, St. Teresa of Avila teaches us that it doesn't hurt to have a sense of humor, even when trying to dodge life's curveballs. We don't have to be absent of pain to be productive, joyful, open to life, or fruitful! Seven years into it, no pregnancy, and I am lacking absolutely *nothing*. On the contrary, my life is bursting with new life.

CHAPTER 7

Why Not IVF?

"Love to be real, it must cost—it must hurt—it must empty us of self."
— *Saint Theresa of Calcutta*

WHEN I WAS IN THE worst of it, I never imagined how fruitful and joyful my life could be without children; without even one pregnancy. There is a deep yearning in all of our hearts to give of ourselves and there is more than one way for that to be satisfying. Sometimes we donate ourselves to little humans, sometimes to bigger humans, and sometimes to both. Sometimes just to bigger humans. I would eventually uncover the great satisfaction in sharing myself with others, but I also felt a specific desire to give myself to a small human. That is how I knew I was called to be a parent even though we were still infertile after all the restorative medical help.

Infertile couples have two options at this point:
- Adopt
- Invest in an artificial reproductive technology.

The way in which we choose to pursue parenthood matters. It requires a sometimes painfully honest reflection of ourselves. Are we being motivated by a love of others and a desire to give ourselves or a disordinate love of self and a desire to receive? It is a difficult question to impose on oneself when attempting to manage a situation that already feels impossibly hard.

If you recall the Harvard Medical School comparative study I mentioned in the Introduction, you might remember how it determined that, "The infertile women had global symptom scores equivalent to the cancer, cardiac rehabilitation and hypertension patients…" This jarring life circumstance tugs mercilessly on a wound shaped by the nagging absence of something that is *very* good and comes *very* easily to almost *everyone* around us. It should come as no surprise that so many couples who are unable to procreate perceive Artificial Reproductive Technologies (ART) to be a merciful opportunity. And it is vital that we remain sensitive to those who maintain such perceptions.

I've considered every aspect of IUI and IVF. Although I understand the beautiful, innate, and even intense desire to have a child, these options have never appealed to me because, frankly, I believe that women and couples deserve better. Chris and I do not feel "bound" by the Catholic Church's firm stance in opposition of it as a life-giving option, but appreciate it because we understand it.

Before I explain why, I want to acknowledge that it is understandable that the idea that anyone might oppose such "amazing" scientific advancements may initially come across as appalling, or at least very confusing, to some. The fact that this Religion advises against it as seriously sinful is either ignored, unknown, or believed to be untrue by many. This will boggle your mind unless these options are fully unpacked, as IUI and IVF are *not* as straightforward as they might seem.

ART introduces a multifaceted topic with many dimensions that are often left unconsidered by the average infertile couple––and by the average person politely recommending it to their struggling friends and/or acquaintances. I can understand why many couples are grateful for ART *and* that it is out of love that some suggest that infertile couples go that route. But I think that only someone who is not aware of all aspects of the process would ask such of anyone.

If it were free and a healthy pregnancy could be guaranteed, Chris and I would still decline for several reasons. This stance is not meant to minimize the pain of infertility, but to acknowledge that it would not serve us as advertised. It's not that the emotional pain associated with the longing to bear a child has disappeared, but its effects have largely been muffled by the recognition of *what God has actually called us to.*

Still, many *understandably* beg the question: "Why don't you just try IVF?"

This seems to be the golden nugget on many inquiring minds. Before I dive into my multifaceted response, let's define some terms so we're all on the same page. There are several procedures that fall under the category of Artificial

Reproductive Technologies, but the most popular are the following:

IUI= Intrauterine Insemination- A man masturbates to obtain semen which a physician inserts into a woman's uterus with hopes that fertilization and implantation will occur; often attempted prior to IVF (more inexpensive and less effective).
IVF= In Vitro Fertilization- A man masturbates to obtain semen which is then combined with a previously

obtained egg to fertilize it. This all takes place in a lab, and then some of the embryos are transferred to the woman's uterus in hopes that pregnancy will occur (expensive). Others are frozen and sometimes destroyed. Multiple attempts are usually required.

Chris and I personally only needed one moral reason to decline these options, despite what our desires did or did not implore. However, I think the desire for IVF has been absent because our decision *not* to use any kind of ART was the result of multiple different practical and emotional reasons in addition to the moral ones.

Please Explain
Even when infertility hurt the most, it was good to see women graduate from hopelessness to pregnancy. But no one can promise *me* that—no friend, acquaintance, doctor, diet, or speaker. The one infertility workshop we went to in Baton Rouge was very well done, but the only woman speaker and author who dealt with infertility eventually got pregnant multiple times and that was her glory story, making me feel as though a pregnancy should solve my problems. These women are able to communicate great truths and words of encouragement to those of us who are still struggling, but it is tempting to imply that, "it'll happen for all of us" or "just hang in there," as if having a baby should be my ultimate goal. I couldn't have put words to it at the time, but that wasn't the message of healing my heart was longing for.

Infertility is not only the denial of a biological child, but the painful denial of my own will. Pregnancy and subsequent birth may, physically, "cure" infertility, but it does not address the brokenness and longing residing within the heart of the one whom, for whatever reason, has been told "no" by God.

This is the empty promise of ART, whose professionals may have good intentions, but subtly suggest that their science will cure, or fill, the gap in my heart. But there is so much more happening than the inability to get pregnant! Pregnancy may not be happening, but *something* is. I longed to be used for a purpose and I didn't immediately recognize that this was the specific route God was calling me to navigate through to discover that/those purpose(s). Scripture insists that suffering bears fruit. Romans 5: 3-5 (NABRE) says, *"...but we even boast of our afflictions, knowing that affliction produces endurance, [4] and endurance, proven character, and proven character, hope, [5] and hope does not disappoint, because the love of God has been poured out into our hearts through the holy Spirit that has been given to us."*

There's only one person who can give me a peace that surpasses all understanding (Philippians 4:7) and he doesn't carry a stethoscope or a lab coat. He did carry the weight of the world on a cross on his back though, and He did it like a champ. ART entices with an escape from suffering, but what I actually needed was to walk through my suffering with my Creator. I wish I would have understood the simple value of the suffering itself sooner! I am even a little offended at the notion that I will not find peace unless I acquire the pregnancy I so ardently desire.

I am a lot more than a woman with parts designed to grow a baby.

I wanted to hear from the woman who never got pregnant and was *still* okay! If I can't learn to accept God's will and trust in Him above all else, a baby won't solve my problems or fully restore my peace. It may please me temporarily, but hopelessness will find me in another way. The desire to have a baby *is* very good. The desire to trust God, even when he doesn't give me the exact thing I am asking for, is better.

I completely understand that seemingly impossible feeling of helplessness which facilitates the desire to take advantage of such a "wonderful" opportunity. But that *feeling* of helplessness where we give God control is where He does His best work! ART becomes a not-so-easy way out of doing the hard work of discovering the fullness of whom God has created us to be. Continuing to peel back the layers with a fine-tooth comb reveals little "wonder" in this option, for me.

I'm Listening...

Above all else, our knowledge that IVF requires the creation of multiple embryos (at least in the large majority of cases), some of which will be frozen, destroyed, or "selectively reduced" is enough. Every embryo is a precious new life—our very own sons and daughters. That means something to me. It will not fill this void to sacrifice the lives of *any* of our children for *any* reason. And if I am not ok with the potential that using hormonal birth control carries to end the life of a newly-conceived baby, then I can't be ok with it here when it would be convenient for me either.

God has designed an incredible process for the transmission of new life. If that makes me sound kind of nerdy about it, it's because I am kind of nerdy about it. Often when man and woman unite during a certain time in a woman's cycle, the ultimate Physician breathes life into every soul. It is a miracle whenever sperm meets egg, whether a couple struggles with fertility or not. The designed process of unity which brings new life into existence is part of what makes it so profound. Keeping the connection between sex and new life intact exhibits a reverence for each, where the child becomes the miraculous result of two complete self-donations of mother and father. Any other way for sperm and egg to unite would be cold and impersonal—not in God's prescription for married love and the co-creation of new life.

But not everyone agrees. If you are one who struggles with the Catholic Church's position on this matter, please consider the exact words She uses to clarify her stance:

CCC (Catechism of the Catholic Church)[16] 2377 explains: *"...Techniques involving only the married couple (homologous artificial insemination and fertilization) are perhaps less reprehensible, yet remain morally unacceptable. They dissociate the sexual act from the procreative act. The act which brings the child into existence is no longer an act by which two persons give themselves to one another, but one that 'entrusts the life and identity of the embryo into the power of doctors and biologists and establishes the domination of technology over the origin and destiny of the human person. Such a relationship of domination is in itself contrary to the dignity and equality that must be common to parents and children.'*

'Under the moral aspect procreation is deprived of its proper perfection when it is not willed as the fruit of the conjugal act, that is to say, of the specific act of the spouses' union . . . . Only respect for the link between the meanings of the conjugal act and respect for the unity of the human being make possible procreation in conformity with the dignity of the person."

According to this, IUI and IVF are not so much merciful options as they are disruptions to the principles of human dignity. The Church is not opposed to ART in an effort to exert authority, or as the result of insensitivity, but out of profound respect for each human person and the dignity of the sacred act of intercourse and the marriage vocation itself. Sex reverences the conception of a human who deserves the dignity of being conceived as the result of the loving sexual embrace of husband and wife.

In the difficulty of the situation, it's easy to unintentionally elevate the goal of a baby above all else. Making the *end* the priority makes it easy to lose sight of the effects of the *means*.

The "no" to IVF initially sounds harsh because, again, the desires that provoke the question being asked in the first place are very good! It is not a response of superiority or out of a lack of understanding of the heart of suffering, but out of love, which if you remember, often hurts. The answer to any question in life will always *be love* or *for love* or *with love*. The ultimate goal of every human life is to reach heaven, basking in eternal glory with Christ who is also known as Love itself. Every human action, whether we recognize it or not, is a God-given exercise to foster growth in that four letter word. What kind of growth doesn't require sacrifice? It is a load on a muscle that causes it to bulk up. It is adding miles to a run that increases endurance. It is denying ourselves the extra calories to lose the extra pounds. It is carving out time for prayer that draws us closer to His Sacred Heart. It is acknowledging God's *"not right now"* as an invitation to learn how to love by our willing self-sacrifice of complying with His will.

The *ways* by which we grow in love is a specific reflection of our uniqueness. It is good that we are not all the same with no individual state in life being superior to another. Our paths to holiness are different, but the vehicle by which we arrive is the same *love*. God's design of intercourse where the two become one is a call to love whether the act results in new human life or not. Many will learn to love through the growth of an embryo and the particular self-sacrifice required in those individual paths. Many others will learn to love through the specific self-sacrifice of acceptance and exploration of another call to fruitfulness when there is no embryo. God knows the best course for growth for each unique soul and desires our ultimate joy perhaps more than we do for ourselves. I believe that re-routing the path to conception would be more of an exhibit of my pride than my ability to sit in the growing pains of love.

It is the unity of the three (God, man, and woman) and no one else that is hallmark to His design, and I'm okay with that. It is a pretty amazing design! It deserves a certain amount of awe and reverence which shouldn't change just because it's not happening for us. If we are going to conceive, it will be the result of sex with my husband. And if we don't, we will *know* it was a small part of God's plan because we have invited him into every moment, especially the most intimate.

But Science…
Yes, God has blessed humans with great intelligence to be able to accomplish some impressive feats like Artificial Reproductive Technologies. He has gifted mankind with incredible knowledge which he can choose to do great things with or exploit for his own purposes, but "With great power comes great responsibility" (I like to quote Spiderman's Grandpa), and plenty of examples in history prove that the very fact that we *can* do something does *not* automatically mean that we should. Go ahead and ask Adam and Eve. Something so precious as the creation of new life warrants some in-depth reflection and consideration with respect to God who is flawless in his *original* intentions and designs.

Go back and re-read the definitions of IUI and IVF. For me, it sounds like a miserably cold imposition on an already emotionally difficult situation. We are talking about the creation of new life which is intended to be the product of love, and the very purpose of ART is to separate conception from unity of spouses. Thanks to the wisdom of the Theology of the Body, we understand that we are made in the image and likeness of God. The Trinity is a constant and never-ending exchange of perfect love. God the Father initiates the gift of life and love to the Son. The Son receives that gift and reciprocates it back to the Father. This exchange of love is so dynamic and so profound, that it creates another Being! It becomes the third Person of the Blessed Trinity, the Holy Spirit.

In like form, man initiates the gift of himself, the gift of life and love, to his wife. She receives that gift and reciprocates it back to her husband. That exchange of love is so dynamic and so profound, that sometimes we give it a name nine months later. Many times that exchange doesn't result in the creation of a new physical being like we hope, but it always carries the ability to produce new life in other fulfilling ways. ***Always.***

Regardless, IUI and IVF babies exist and have **equal value and worth** as babies conceived naturally, babies conceived out of wedlock, and babies conceived from rape. Each pregnancy which results from premarital sex or rape, for example, contains a baby whose dignity is no different than a baby conceived by a consenting married couple. But that doesn't make the circumstances that caused the pregnancy favorable, or even okay, for any of the parties involved. God respects the laws of nature as he designed them and always allows good to come out of situations and decisions he has *not* ordained. Man has the intelligence to create a gun which he has the free will to use to harm someone if he chooses. The laws of nature ordain a bullet to penetrate flesh whether it was used with "good intentions" or not.

The reality is that God does not need a lab and physicians to create new life. If pregnancy doesn't happen with respect to the way *He* invented it, I'm going to pay closer attention to what other beautiful things he may have in store for us. *Because* ART was not an option for us, I began to take an honest look at the things that were only happening in our lives because we couldn't get pregnant—things I would never trade! More on that soon...

But Speaking of Science...
His invention involves multiple incredible and appropriately-timed processes taking place within the woman's body cyclically to prepare for a conception that most of the time doesn't happen (I know. My nerd is showing again). Every biological action has a special and important purpose. I think this gives us a glimpse into how precious God views new life. So, if a pregnancy is not occurring, we should try to figure out why. As I dove into learning about the woman's body, I realized that it would often be either counterproductive or ineffective to bypass many of these processes to essentially force a pregnancy **despite** the woman's body screaming that at least one of these processes is not working correctly.

For example: A fever is not a disease in and of itself. It is a part of an incredible design intended to alert us to an underlying problem that needs to be addressed. Well, a woman's body is designed to achieve pregnancy under normal conditions. When that doesn't happen, there is a reason. One of the most valuable pieces of women's health information I have acquired is that infertility is *not* a disease, but a symptom of some abnormality within her system. Fertility/ovulation/the menstrual cycle is a sign of health which some refer to as the fifth vital sign. ART, even when successful, never restores a woman's health. And I deserve better than that—all women do.

This way of looking at my system has also helped me *not* to feel so much more broken and inadequate than the rest of humanity who *is* making babies. Infertility is not a reflection of who I am or the result of something I have done wrong. It is not an inability to become fully woman, or even fully a mother. There are countless abnormalities that can exist within the human body that affect some individuals' ability to do just about anything. I have one that somehow impedes conception and/or healthy implantation of new life.

Restoring function to the woman's body, however, is a goal I think everyone can get behind, but many are not aware that it is an option. If a woman's hormone levels are balanced and monitored naturally as an aspect of general health (not a part of ART and rarely a part of mainstream gynecology), if she has a healthy diet, if she is aware of the connection between fertility and overall health, and if she has had adequate restorative surgical techniques (if applicable) by a specialist using anti-adhesion measures, she will be more likely to conceive naturally *and* more likely to maintain that pregnancy to full term.

The keywords here are "more likely," not "absolutely and without fail." However, even when pregnancy is never achieved, many women will experience a relief of associated symptoms and some **knowledge** of the cause—like me. If optimal health and knowledge of body is the ultimate desire of the woman, it is possible for her to feel some satisfaction through the experience even if a baby does not result. If we can shift our ultimate focus to health in this respect, a woman is less likely to experience such drastic disappointment because health is something that can always improve, providing some kind of result.

This type of healthcare is available through Creighton Model charting (CreightonModel.com and fertilitycare. org) and NaProTechnology (Naprotechnology.com). NaPro is 1.5-3 times more effective than IVF and at a fraction of the cost; almost always covered by insurance. You can also find Restorative Reproductive Medical Professionals at www.femmhealth.com, www. mycatholicdoctor.com, and www.fabmbase.org.

NaProTechnology is not the only brand of medicine that seeks to restore a woman's health. Fortunately, *Restorative Reproductive Medicine* is a growing branch of medicine housing many healthcare providers who don't prescribe birth control or recommend ART in hopes of addressing underlying problems. I have several Creighton clients who have come to me for instruction after having a failed ART experience, and all are shocked and pleased by the amount of information their chart and NaPro medical consultant are able to provide them within a matter of months after seeing a reproductive endocrinologist for years. What a relief it is to be able to remove those first two letters from *un*explained infertility!

This type of medicine does not serve us as a magical "pill," so to speak, or miracle fix. I ***don't*** recommend attempting to *"fix"* friends and relatives by offering this alternative to them as such. The overall purpose is to expand the knowledge of women of all ages, ideally starting with teens, about fertility awareness so that they are aware of how a normal reproductive system functions and are able to confront arising health issues early, maintaining ideal health and fertility as they age.

This *Fertility Appreciation* will allow young women *and men* to approach marriage and potential pregnancies in the best position possible. You can find some excellent resources on this topic, a comparison of methods that foster fertility appreciation, and solidarity at *www.fabmbase.org*, *www.managingyourfertility.com*, and *www.totalwhine.com*.

I am not suggesting that this shift of perspective will make women immune to any sense of defeat or sadness associated with infertility. I am advocating for an understanding of infertility as a (or one of many) symptom(s) of some range of potential underlying dysfunctions in a woman's body––not the result of a moral error or proof of insufficiency as a woman, Catholic, or daughter of God. The desire to have a baby is innately beautiful, but our physical, emotional, psychological, spiritual, and marital health are, actually, more important and need to be intact in order to be content, *and* to raise a baby well. It is often devastating when a baby doesn't come, but staunchly pursuing those five health goals will undoubtedly and without fail provide results that **will** satisfy your heart and mind to great capacity.

Cost
I can't open up this conversation without discussing cost. And I'm not just talking about the financial kind.

"The next step was IUI because I wanted a baby... it ended up being one of the worst experiences of my life. I don't want to over dramatize it—it was more of an emotional experience than a physical (although it was very uncomfortable). Going through that experience aligned the teachings of the Church for me...the Catholic Church opposes it...and going through it (on a spiritual

level), I now know why. It's hard to explain...I was in a really bad place after that, even before we got the results back."
-Julie Liberto, one time IUI patient

This was a quote from a young woman I interviewed after she finally got answers about her health and infertility via her new NaPro doctor whom she discovered shortly after this failed IUI experience. I was engaging in a conversation with her about Polycystic Ovarian Syndrome (PCOS) and was unaware that she attempted IUI and was shocked by the way she described this other aspect of ART. The high financial cost of IVF is common knowledge, but you don't often hear of the potential drastic emotional costs involved with the process—as if infertility alone wasn't emotional enough.

Can you imagine? If what I am saying about ART being outside of God's plan for the creation of new life is true, can you imagine going to such great and painful lengths to reach a different goal than the ones He is just waiting for us to ask Him about? Including goals for improved health? I have experienced too much goodness through being exactly where I am at each step of infertility to trade any of it.

Financial cost is one of the most obvious roadblocks to many in this situation. A simple Google search will tell you the average price tag for *one* (uno, une) round of IVF is between $10-15,000 and that doesn't include the cost of medication which can run as high as $3,000 and is not usually covered by insurance. Honestly, that is a lot cheaper than I expected. I imagine that it is not unusual for the price to increase even more so.

Another simple Google search will tell you that you should try for at least three IVF cycles, so do the math. There is no guarantee that any individual round will result in pregnancy or reach full term because the underlying causes are usually unknown. According to *Medical Express*[7], "Overall, for women starting IVF, 33% have a baby as a result of their first cycle, increasing to 54-77% by the eighth cycle." The eighth cycle of physical, financial, and emotional stress. And the chances decrease as we age. Many women/couples will pay this amount more than once, investing more and more money, time, and emotions into a goal that may never be reached. What stress might that put on an individual? A Marriage?

That is the part that often feels impossible. Despite our very best intentions and efforts, a baby is often not the end result. This lack of control feels like an assault against our very womanhood because, again, the desire for a baby is very good. It is how God created us! But I would challenge you not to view this lack of control as such a bad and inescapable fate. It is an uncomfortable position God allows while waiting for us to reach out and choose *His* hand, which is patiently awaiting our grasp so He can overwhelm us with His love and shower us with *His* gifts. They are real. He is real. What if we stepped into that instead of trying to take charge?

There is no doubt that infertility is an unexpected life circumstance that deserves attention. But not *just any* attention will do. We deserve so much more than what ART has to offer. Now that I have elaborated on that very topic, let me give you a short, but comprehensive review of my responses to that infamous question "Why not use Artificial Reproductive Technologies?"

IUI & IVF:
1) Both circumvent God's perfect design for the co-creation of new life, separating procreation from the sexual act, and undermining human dignity.
2) Both circumvent the underlying health issue(s) preventing conception.
3) Both can be extremely emotionally invasive (on top of what is already emotionally exhausting).
4) Both can easily make a baby the priority over God and spouse.
5) Both can put undue stress on a marriage.
6) Both can be physically uncomfortable/painful.
7) Neither have guarantees or high success rates.
8) Neither improve health, even when a baby is not the result.
9) Neither continue to support the women throughout pregnancy.

IVF
1) Most often, IVF creates multiple embryos with a low survival rate; many of these new lives are frozen or destroyed. Those would be our sons and daughters––no matter how small.
2) It's very expensive; multiple rounds are often required with no guarantee.

There are many aspects of life that God expects us to exercise control over (ourselves, for example), but the creation of new life is His domain. I am personally grateful for that. He chooses to bring new life into the world in about a million different ways in addition to delivering babies. And this is what I am continuing to discover more and more with each day. There are no limitations to God's goodness. What if I were to miss out on what He is truly calling me to do because I have been so focused on a goal I made for myself, rather than the one He made for me? For my husband?

If we had focused on ART, I would have avoided accepting myself for how God made me. And I'm pretty awesome. We would have missed out on the incredible things He specifically created us to do, which I cannot wait to tell you about!

CHAPTER 8

Spiritual Freaking Motherhood

"If you are what you should be, you will set the whole world ablaze!"
— *Saint Catherine of Sienna*

MY MOM IS AN INCREDIBLE giver. I have never known anyone to be as selfless and serving as the woman who gave me my name—even to her own detriment. She takes care of her family and home until she is literally falling asleep on the sofa from wearing herself out. And boy, does she have an imagination! Our birthday parties and daily activities sparkled with her creativity throughout childhood. Now our children get that privilege.

Even as an adult, I don't have to lift a finger when visiting because all of my needs *and* wants are fulfilled by her without me asking and without complaint. I have to make an effort to contribute more so that I don't accidentally take advantage of her. And don't even get me started on how she becomes even super-er mom when we are sick!

I think we all know what her love language is.

She also has a huge heart that beats for the Church. She feels like she was created to teach Bible School and she soars in that role. Teaching Confirmation and Religion classes, helping with youth group, chaperoning retreats, keeping everyone in line with Church teaching, you name it, she thrives at it. Her spiritual motherhood is an incredible gift to the world.

My momma was no stranger to suffering, either. She was blessed with three live births, but also had three miscarriages. At forty years old, and five years after I was born, her doctor felt a relatively large mass inside of her during a routine checkup. He scheduled surgery two weeks later, fearing it was cancerous. It ended up being a rare benign tumor about the size of a small orange on her cervix, which he removed along with her uterus. She went into surgery thinking he may remove an ovary and woke up with a hysterectomy. She already had myself, my brother, and my sister, so that softened a blow that would've been shockingly devastating.

At the time, NaProTechnology wasn't as easily accessible and she often wonders if her fertility might have been saved had she had access to this modern and restorative approach to healthcare. Nonetheless, her three babies were and are precious to her and this has been reflected in her gift of self-donation throughout all of our lives. It was always clear to us that staying at home and raising her children was extremely important to her. She would always say, "I'd stay at home to raise y'all even if it meant we could only afford to eat peanut butter and jelly sandwiches."

"Mrs. G," as her students called her, has been quite fruitful.

I am blessed with two devout and caring parents who worked hard to give us everything we needed. And although I was made by God to be incredibly fruitful like every other human being on the planet, I am not called to bear fruit in the same exact ways as many who have gone before me. I've quite literally tried and failed––or at least it felt like I had failed. There was some unspoken message residing in my bones that I should mirror my life to the Catholic norm, or at least my perception of such. Whether directly spoken or not, there was an *expected* way of doing things: get married, have children, quit job to stay at home (change in job, really), have more children, etc.

My parents had perfect intentions and handed on exceptional values to me and my siblings. They passed on to us what they knew and experienced as faithful Catholics. At the time, part of that consisted of coloring within the lines of that important sequence. And that message really wasn't any different than what I was receiving at church. There was little to no emphasis on NFP outside the intention to avoid pregnancy (fertility awareness), infertility, alternatives to IVF, adoption, or the beauty of spiritual parenthood and fruitfulness outside of bearing biological children. There was little encouragement to be open to and explore *all* the gifts God has given me, even the ones that seem unconventional.

I think this is an unintended side effect of the (necessary) fight for life in opposition to abortion and contraception and praise of large families when it's *not balanced* with an appreciation of the worth of each individual regardless of their ability to achieve and maintain a pregnancy. As time passed, I recognized a growing desire to be drawn more into my parish community by being assured that I was equally capable of bearing fruit as my fertile counterparts. Infertile couples need to feel the embrace of their Church despite their apparent inability to conceive a child! Fertile couples are starving for permission to explore their God-given gifts that complement their physical motherhood. Subtle implications and overt statements and actions, although unintended, have caused me to feel viewed as inferior to other Catholic women and couples who bear children. It has been very isolating within the Church that I love.

You see, I typically follow instructions really well. But I have a very limited amount of control over the ability to achieve a pregnancy. When it didn't happen, I felt like a failure in my ability to be fruitful and do "what I was created to do" or "what Catholic women are supposed to do" as defined by the living faithful around me. I continued on that downward spiral of monthly failure feeling helpless and hopeless until I stopped ignoring that tiny voice inside of me crying out to be used for *some* purpose; *my* purpose. How does **God** define womanhood? Motherhood?

I remember standing in the shower one day (why do so many moments of great inspiration happen in the shower?) having one of many pow-wows with my Maker and internally taking another tiny step closer towards acceptance as He called me forward.

"Okay, God, I accept this cross of infertility today. I'll try again tomorrow. But please give me purpose. Please make use of my suffering! I have such a great desire to give myself as a mother! Please fill this void."

We all desire to be of use and serve a purpose. The better we understand ourselves in light of whom God says we are, the more of use we become. Part of the reason infertility beats up on us so much is because one of our purposes as women is built into our very bodies and it's not functioning! The absences of a baby bump and a child are obvious as we simply walk out into public spaces and look around, heck - who needs to walk outside? Just turn on the TV or open up your social media pages. They are everywhere. Having babies is most certainly a beautiful purpose–that's why this is so painful–but it is far from the only purpose and far from a superior one. It is the same for any other cause for feelings of inadequacy. God ultimately wants what is best for us. Asking him for my purpose was hard, and not only essential to healing from infertility, but essential to getting to know myself.

As a ranking member of the "Rule Follower" club, it was easy to imagine being perceived as a failure by my Creator when I "broke" what I thought was a cardinal rule of following "the Catholic norm." However, my request to serve another purpose (since I had been unable to bear children) was not received by Him as an inconvenience or as subordinate, but with great anticipation and excitement; as if he was a doting parent on Christmas morning just waiting for His child to open up *countless* priceless gifts that were selected just for me. It was never about what others thought I should do with my life, or even about what I *thought* I wanted, but what God created me for.

When I asked Him to give my suffering purpose, I felt the relief of His reassuring voice: *"I was hoping you'd ask..."*

Defining *"mother"*
I used to hear the term "spiritual parenthood" and brush it off as if the concept was only somewhat meaningful, barely important enough to give a second thought to–– like a consolation prize. But where would we be without the spiritual motherhood of the Blessed Mother or Mother

Teresa? What about the fatherhood of amazing priests who counsel, console, and offer the Sacraments for us? It doesn't consist of some boring deed you do 'cuz you have to or 'cuz you want to get brownie points.

It's *spiritual freaking motherhood*, it's needed, and it's a big deal!

Have you comforted a friend when they have felt incredible sorrow? Have you given direction to anyone in need? Have you listened to someone's heart? Have you cooked for someone or given them a much needed hug? Have you prayed for anyone? Have you used your creativity? Have you used any of the unique gifts God has given you to make the world better?

Then I tell you that you have, indeed, not only been a mother or father, but a much needed and valued one.

In Pope St. John Paul II's *Mulieris Dignitatum*[15], He explains:
"Does not Jesus bear witness to this reality when he answers the exclamation of that woman in the crowd who blessed him for Mary's motherhood: 'Blessed is the womb that bore you, and the breasts that you sucked!'? Jesus replies: 'Blessed rather are those who hear the word of God and keep it' (Lk 11:27-28). Jesus confirms the meaning of motherhood in reference to the body, but at the same time he indicates an even deeper meaning, which is connected with the order of the spirit: it is a sign of the Covenant with God who 'is spirit' (Jn 4: 24). This is true above all for the motherhood of the Mother of God. The motherhood of every woman, understood in the light of the Gospel, is similarly not only 'of flesh and blood': it expresses a profound 'listening to the word of the living God' and a readiness to 'safeguard' this Word, which is 'the word of eternal life' (cf. Jn 6:68)."

There is a profound beauty in the biological connection of mother and child. But as demonstrated by Jesus in the reference above, an even deeper meaning of motherhood is exhibited in a woman's ability to safeguard the Word of God and transmit it to humanity, whether stemming from her own biology or not, or both!

The Apostolic Letter[15] repeatedly expands on the widespread presence and value of spiritual motherhood: *"Moreover, contemplating Mary's mysterious sanctity, imitating her charity, and faithfully fulfilling the Father's will, the Church herself becomes a mother by accepting God's word in faith. For by her preaching and by baptism she brings forth to a new and immortal life children who are conceived by the Holy Spirit and born of God".[45] This is motherhood "according to the Spirit" with regard to the sons and daughters of the human race."*

Wow.

The desire to be a mother is simply a desire to nurture, love, create, educate, explore, beautify, discipline, comfort, serve, and the list goes on. Every woman is called to be a mother, biological child or not. Every woman has the potential to be fertile because *to be fertile* simply means *to be capable of producing fruit* or *abundantly productive*. We bear fruit when we use the gifts God has given us. That is enough! You are enough. A large amount of my healing was derived by using my gifts for the purposes for which He created me––and my husband.

The same goes for every man. We call priests "Father" not because they have biological children, but because they have a fatherly role as a visible reflection of our Heavenly Father on earth. They are incredibly life-giving. But not every good Catholic man is called to be a priest, a husband, and/or a father with biological children. We *are* all called to be open to life.

Then there is our amazing, immaculate, and stunning picture of perfection, Mother Mary. She is also my very own Patron Saint. In her, we have a radiant example of biological motherhood, but Christ also very specifically entrusted her as spiritual mother to *all of humanity* through some of His last words on the cross:
"Standing by the cross of Jesus were his mother and his mother's sister, Mary the wife of Clopas, and Mary of Magdala. [26] When Jesus saw his mother[b] and the disciple there whom he loved, he said to his mother, "Woman, behold, your son." [27] Then he said to the disciple, "Behold, your mother." And from that hour the disciple took her into his home."(John 19: 25-27, NABRE)

We have been gifted with an extraordinary woman whom we are all privileged to call *mother*. It is through her example that we understand the fullness of our vocation. Ultimately, our dignity is realized through our union with God, not our ability to procreate: *"Thus, by considering the reality 'Woman - Mother of God', we enter in a very appropriate way into this Marian Year meditation [1988]. This reality also determines the essential horizon of reflection on the dignity and the vocation of women. In anything we think, say or do concerning the dignity and the vocation of women, our thoughts, hearts and actions must not become detached from this horizon. The dignity of every human being and the vocation corresponding to that dignity find their definitive measure in union with God[15]."*

Mary is not only an exquisite nurturer and comforter, but she gives us direction and draws us close to her Son in ways that only a mother can. She is the perfect marriage of every single motherly quality intended to love her children on earth–none of which were born from her womb–right into heaven. All women are called to imitate her.

She is the ideal role model for every woman that will ever exist and is someone to whom two of my closest friends, Elise and Lisa, have always looked up to. Neither have children and are some of the most fertile and fruitful people I know. One is infertile with one miscarriage and now they both have a serious medical reason to avoid pregnancy. God doesn't consider us any less valuable to our families or the world because we are unable to conceive––or *until* we are able to conceive. Every human is cherished and every human carries a cross––probably a few. It is a matter of *how* God has designed us to bear fruit. Sometimes it is obvious, but sometimes discovering our purpose(s) is the result of being stretched and molded into a better version of ourselves.

"The present reflections, now at an end, have sought to recognize, within the "gift of God", what he, as Creator and Redeemer, entrusts to women, to every woman. In the Spirit of Christ, in fact, women can discover the entire meaning of their femininity and thus be disposed to making a "sincere gift of self" to others, thereby finding themselves." -Mulieris Dignitatum[15]

Infertility causes us to raise many questions about ourselves, highlighting what we lack. Just as it is with any limiting factor or situation that ruptures our expectations, the challenge remains to make a sincere gift of ourselves to Christ; to others. When we are able to do this, no matter the circumstance, we are able to truly discover the person He created us to be.

Purpose

A couple of years ago, I heard Jennifer Fulwiler give a talk at the "Abiding Together Conference" in Lafayette, Louisiana, on this idea of "your blue flame," which she has since released a best-selling book about. She explained that your blue flame is *that thing* that God has created you to do to make the world better. I interpret it as our specific and unique gifts and talents. She goes on to say that it is typically something you enjoy, are good at, and can spend an incredible amount of time doing, but doesn't drain you, it actually gives you energy. The light bulbs began to turn on for me.

John Henry Newman (1801-1890) wrote: *"God has created me to do him some definite service; he has committed some work to me which he has not committed to another. I have my mission—I may never know it in this life, but I shall be told it in the next. I am a link in a chain, a bond of connection between persons. He has not created me for nothing. Therefore, I will trust him. Whatever, wherever I am. I cannot be thrown away."*

Infertile or not, harboring *feelings* of inadequacy or not, all humans have purpose. We all have at least one blue flame; at least one mission: not just to bring new life into the world, but into our individual lives and the lives of others. New life does not *just* come in the form of a bouncing baby girl or boy.

I didn't recognize how fruitful I was before infertility, and the struggle itself gave me fuel to pursue more passions in hopes of bringing meaning to it all. It began with the drive to adopt. Although not every childless couple is called to adoption, that was where God led us. It was only about three months after my "worst day ever" that I was ready to wholeheartedly step into that process with Chris. After that was set in motion, I directed my attention towards what was next most pressing in my heart and well before we were selected by a birthmother: women's health advocacy.

Over the years, I had recognized that my infertility was most likely a result of an extremely late medical diagnosis due to a devastating lack of women's health education for women of all ages. By the time I discovered the authentic and restorative healthcare approach of NaProTechnology, it was apparently too late to help me achieve a pregnancy but not too late to give me some answers, drastically improve my symptoms, and point other women in the right direction *before* it becomes an issue for them: thus, the birth of my "Taking Back the Terms" outreach. Now known as @whitelotusbloming, and with the addition of a non-profit organization called @fabmbase that I co-founded with a close friend, I'm reaching the masses on social media, through videos, and via public speaking, with superior alternatives to birth control and IUI/IVF.

I became a Creighton Model FertilityCare Practitioner who is trained to teach women and couples how to monitor and maintain their own reproductive and gynecological health. Although I am able to serve women in all reproductive categories, the Creighton Model offers the specific benefit of identifying early risk factors for infertility and providing access to NaProTechnology physicians. I have become an important step in the process of helping other women to become pregnant who may have otherwise been unable to, but most importantly, to improve their health.

The experience of my first infertile client achieving a pregnancy was profoundly special—especially after reading the email in which she shared the good news with me: *"...two days before that I took a pregnancy test and I'm pregnant!! I'm twelve weeks now and we are so excited! I've been meaning to reach out to you for a while to thank you so much for everything. You were a listening ear, shoulder to cry on, and a wealth of knowledge. I can never thank you enough for your support. I hope you've had a lot of success stories and that you know you're doing great things! Thank you!!!"*

Helping others tends to be an uplifting purpose for the average human being, whether we are suffering or not. We all also need a cathartic outlet for relieving our emotions. I began blogging immediately, which came as a surprise to me because I never enjoyed writing until I had something so important to express. A couple of years after I started writing, I explored my gifts further by attempting to write lyrics to accompany my *unconventional* passion for rapping. Recording and performing has fed my soul and my faith in ways that wouldn't have been possible without infertility.

"*Holy Family*,*" a song I co-wrote with International speaker and rapper Oscar TwoTen:*
When my heart's cut deep and bleeding out on the floor
The meaning of family's knocking on death's door
I need the comfort of my mother who is calling my name
Different womb—but she loves me the same
Can't see they're looking at your Son from afar
So many are missing out on the gift that you are
Crushing Satan's head; repeat
Baby blue–packing spiritual heat
Best combination of delicate and fierce
You are stronger than ever, with your own flesh pierced
Giving birth to my King I will never forget it
You are flawless...and taking none of the credit.
Beauty–unaware. True finesse.
You gave that angel your infamous "Yes!"
Trusted by the very Author of mankind
It was your bulletproof faith prompting His first sign
You triggered counting to His final hour

You show us how to suffer with grace–God's power
I'm selfish. I can't understand–how seamless your desires are with I AM
Dying to self–like you, to Him I run
Like a mirror you reflect the perfect longings of your Son
Motherhood perfected like none we have seen
Mrs. B, step aside, and honor the real Queen...

That last line is a dig at Beyonce who is often referred to as "Queen B" and has taken photographs that tastelessly suggest a comparison between the two "queens." Rapping began as an expressive outlet for the deep pain I have felt, but progressed to other topics close to my heart. It gives me the ability to speak passionately to many truths.

More Purpose
Nearly five years into our marriage, Chris and I were trained as a marriage prep mentor couple, which became another incredible blessing in our lives and marriage. We never planned on adding this ministry to our tool belt, but discerned it would be one of the many ways God would call us to be fruitful in our marriage after friends of ours got engaged and asked us to prepare them. Knowledge gained from this experience has truly enriched our own marriage and blessed us with another dimension of true *parenthood*.

I was unaware of it at the time, but something amazing was happening as we discussed a significant experience that took place in the lives of our most recent engaged couple. I received a text the next day from the future bride: "Hey I just wanted to let you know––I was talking with [my fiance] and I asked him how he was liking marriage prep. He said how much he really liked you and Chris. He then was saying, I really liked what Mary was saying about [the situation we discussed]. He was like, 'she really broke through to me, like my mom wouldn't be able to do that. She was just really real and got through to me.' I just thought how good of a mother you are…that to [my fiance], he was able to feel that motherly sense from you, and I wanted to just let you know that!! You're a great mom, Mary!!!"

I was deeply touched! I knew God had been using Chris and I to communicate the beauty of the Sacrament as a marriage prep mentor couple, but it never occurred to me that I might be used as a mother—and impact this couple so significantly.

My first vocations are wife to Chris and mother to Bella, but when I have extra time, I can share myself in the other ways for which I have been created. I can see now why God has not called us, personally, to have a home full of children. And exploring my *other* gifts has allowed me to come alive in new and exciting ways that are healing me from the inside out.

God has given me an innate desire for public speaking, writing, educating, motivating, sharing my faith, caring for my family and friends, rapping, podcasting, making videos, drawing, comforting others, making people laugh, fighting for truth, connecting with others, raising my daughter… and those are only the things I want to do. When they're done as an act of love, even the things I don't feel like doing bear great fruit. Imagine all the different ways that list can be used to make me fertile. The list of my own personal desires is only limited by my willingness to pursue Christ, challenge myself, and appreciate the immeasurable beauty that is within me.

It was my infertility that facilitated the search within myself for whom God created me to be. What is your source of suffering stirring inside of you? What is it teaching you? Even if I didn't always know it in my heart, I knew in my brain that God is good. Not a little bit good, but *very* good. And if he wasn't allowing me to get pregnant, there had to be a really good reason for it. I had numerous gifts I wasn't cultivating or exploring that would have stayed on the shelf, collecting dust, had I not experienced such suffering and longing for more, and had God not loved me enough to say "no."

Neither the purpose(s) of our suffering nor our gifts have to be any grand gesture. It could be something as large-scale as running for President or as seemingly insignificant as growing in empathy, and anywhere in between. Both are important and can have a major impact on ourselves and others.

If to be pregnant is to nurture and grow life and to prepare a loving environment for humans to thrive and flourish into the people God created them to be, then my prayers have not only been answered, but exceeded.

The Biologically Fertile

God calls both man and woman–sick and well, rich and poor, fertile and infertile–to be fruitful; productive; producing good. I recently spoke with a close friend and mother of five who expressed a desire for more in her own life, inquiring about how women can be more of service in the church. She asked a local friend and priest who responded with "women beautify the church." And although many men are absolutely capable and called to do that in their own way, he personally did not think he was able to and was expressing an appreciation for the women around him.

Some will only define "beautifying" the church as providing pleasing aesthetics, and even though that is a worthy and important purpose, stretch your imagination a bit to consider how many different creative ways it can be interpreted. The church is not *just* the building, but the people, and not reserved to a singular geographical location. *"To beautify"* does not just refer to external appearance but to the interior life. You name the gift—the church needs it *and* you.

"While the dignity of woman witnesses to the love which she receives in order to love in return, the biblical "exemplar" of the Woman also seems to reveal the true order of love which constitutes woman's own vocation.

Vocation is meant here in its fundamental, and one may say universal significance, a significance which is then actualized and expressed in women's many different "vocations" in the Church and the world.

The moral and spiritual strength of a woman is joined to her awareness that God entrusts the human being to her in a special way. Of course, God entrusts every human being to each and every other human being. But this entrusting concerns women in a special way–precisely by reason of their femininity–and this in a particular way determines their vocation." -Mulieris Dignitatum[15]

This same friend continued to confide in me about her own hyperfertility, questioning if it was her sole purpose to have babies while feeling the call to more in addition to her beautiful and important role of raising her children. It is ultimately between God and each individual woman/couple to discern individual roles, and how and when to use their gifts and grow their families. No one else can or should answer for her/them.

But could it be possible that he allows hyperfertility in some to foster even greater discipline and self-control at times for some greater reason? Perhaps she *is* being called to bear fruit in a different way at this time. She agreed that this is what she was focusing on during Lent. The important ingredient in any fruitful family recipe is openness to God in frequent discernment, regardless of state in life.

The struggles are different, but they are real for both the fertile and the infertile. I do not put my friend in this category, but it is quite possible to give birth to many children and be barren in regards to fruitfulness.

There are a few unexpected privileges to being an infertile mother (besides not having to recover physically after giving birth), one of which is having the concept of motherhood sliding more naturally into perspective. I think that the true gift of motherhood was more fully realized for me as I began to understand how little control any of us have over it. Women who experience hyperfertility can relate to this as well. It is easy to have the *perception* of control when pregnancy is intentionally achieved during a time of fertility in a woman's cycle, or even without much effort at all. But again, the creation of new life is God's domain. He is still the one to drop that precious soul into every new life.

Our primary identity is as beloved children of God. And although we wear many different important hats throughout life, what and *whom* defines us? It is not our husband, friends, work, nor is it our children. We could contribute nothing of worth to this world and still be inherently valued by God. When biological motherhood is a sole focus whether for the fertile or infertile, it is harder to keep our identity intact. Even the most fertile woman will one day cease having the ability to produce children. What then? If a woman defines herself by her service to her children *alone*, what happens when all the children are grown and leave the house? She may not realize it right away, but her worth has not changed—just like the woman unable to conceive.

Women who are able to bear children are blessed with incredible gifts and talents of which God desires to use in incredible ways to enrich our world in as much as He does for the biologically infertile. One of my many important and treasured roles is mother to our adopted daughter, Bella. My experience and adversity in receiving that title has taught me that I am so much more than *just* a mother to her. I absolutely adore our time together, but I also get excited about conquering the world in my own little ways with my own little talents.

"Therefore the Church gives thanks for each and every woman: for mothers, for sisters, for wives; for women consecrated to God in virginity; for women dedicated to the many human beings who await the gratuitous love of another person; for women who watch over the human persons in the family, which is the fundamental sign of the human community; for women who work professionally, and who at times are burdened by a great social responsibility; for "perfect" women and for "weak" women - for all women as they have come forth from the heart of God in all the beauty and richness of their femininity; as they have been embraced by his eternal love; as, together with men, they are pilgrims on this earth, which is the temporal "homeland" of all people and is transformed sometimes into a "valley of tears" as they assume, together with men, a common responsibility for the destiny of humanity according to daily necessities and according to that definitive destiny which the human family has in God himself, in the bosom of the ineffable Trinity." -Mulieris Dignitatum[15]

God has certainly not only blessed us with a broad and meaningful description of motherhood, but with an incredible Pope and Saint to communicate the reality of these truths so clearly to us. I am grateful for the affirmation of what God has so clearly placed in our hearts, even though we often find it challenging to verbalize *and* to believe that He *really is* that good. There are no limits to God's goodness. Fortunately, Chris and I have both been blessed with loving and *flexible* families who accept us the way we are. Although all of us expected pregnancy to follow marriage at some point like it does for most, we were fully loved and supported as we stumbled through the five stages of grief when it didn't happen. We have been incredibly blessed to have families that have fully embraced our new addition from the start, even though she doesn't share any of our DNA.

You're handmaid–full of grace
Theotokos, y'all make some space!
God of creation your own flesh and blood
Sharing you–woman, behold your son!
Oh you thought motherhood and biology were the same?
Like she doesn't know every single one of our last names?
One with the Spirit and one perfect wife
One with His mission and one with his life
Your living, breathing tabernacle
There is no enemy that you can't tackle
You can find Satan on a thrown giving a hurl
'Cuz he can't take gettin' beat by a girl
To know you is to love you–I can't get enough
God wrote your story, I can't make this stuff up!
Beween you and Joe, there ain't no typical spouse
This ain't just a home, it's a powerhouse!

CHAPTER 9

Her

"Since love grows within you, so beauty grows. For love is the beauty of the soul."
— Saint Augustine

SHE IS A LITTLE CLUMSY and prefers fruity desserts over chocolate ones, just like her daddy. She makes funny faces and loves to draw, like me. She is tiny and dark-skinned with jet black hair like her birth mother. She is nearly three and a half feet of sweet, smiling, princess-loving perfection and we wouldn't have her any other way. We also, quite literally, wouldn't *have our daughter* any other way than through adoption.

It's hard to approach this next topic because I want to do it justice. It's one that is so close to my heart that I get emotional when thinking about the pure joy we receive by the mere presence of our adopted daughter. I can no longer fathom a world where I desire anything–even pregnancy–over the opportunity to wake her up every morning.

Chris was ready to adopt well before I was. He was always open to having both adopted kids and biological children. I envied the freedom he felt in welcoming a new child into our home regardless of whether or not our characteristics would match. But it was also something that was discussed frequently in his home growing up. His mom took a sincere interest in helping women with unplanned pregnancies, and his family knew children who were adopted. His parents had even begun their own process of adoption up until they became pregnant. The whole idea felt more complicated to me. On top of my stereotypical hesitancies, I had an unfounded fear that starting the process meant sealing our fate as infertile, or at least my acceptance of such. I knew that made no sense, but sometimes *thoughts, or beliefs,* are like that. *My* perception was *our* reality.

On my "worst day ever," I made one of those classic "deals" with God for three more months. If we weren't pregnant by then, we would start the adoption process. I realized later that that defined time limit was really just giving me time to begin to heal, accept, and attempt to shift my focus towards something (or someone) outside of myself. I had just done a lot of the heavy lifting by choosing to love my Creator despite feeling completely rejected. It was time to choose to trust Him into this new depth of our relationship. It was a decision I would need to continue to make every day.

Another crucial factor worth mentioning in my ability to move forward with adoption was Chris's incredible patience with me. He waited for about a year for me to be ready *without* nagging me, giving me the freedom I needed to address my internal conflict. God was the only One who could get me to the right place at the right time and He provided the grace Chris needed to *do nothing* but support me. Sometimes the holiest thing we can do is *nothing* but wait patiently.

This was not easy for either of us, but few things of great worth are. The three months passed and I would stick to my word, which gave me relief from running away from what God was asking of me. I felt like Julia Roberts in "Runaway Bride." She invested herself as a fiancée to three different men––all good people, but none were right as her future spouse. With each failed relationship, she became what she thought others wanted while unaware of what and whom she was called to. Even her egg preference changed with each man––it went from "scrambled, salt, pepper, and dill" to "egg whites" to "poached, like me."

Then Richard Gere's character comes along to write an article on her, the *runaway bride*, and, as he begins to see her for who she is, he challenges her to do the same. She was livid, but she was also attracted to his authenticity and began the hard work of discovering herself. This gave her the freedom to take many different leaps of faith. She finally pursued her gift of crafting and sold her artwork, figured out which style of eggs she favored, and eventually tied the knot.

It wasn't just that I was running away from adoption. I was avoiding the beautiful truth about myself as God made me because I had been so focused on my own goals, and I needed to discover myself, too.

I *had* to combine my love for analogies and this movie for the perfect "I'm ready to adopt a baby with you" announcement to Chris. I hadn't told him about my wait-three-months plan, so he had no idea it was coming. And just like Julia Roberts did at the end of my all-time favorite Rom Com, I put my running shoes in a box and handed them to Chris on one special night. This was one of the very few nights I wiped tears from his eyes as we slow-danced in front of the end screen of the movie. True story.

Although we would continue to try and get pregnant, I honestly never looked back after making the decision to start the process because I was absolutely sure of three things at this point:
- God was calling us to be parents now or soon
- We couldn't get pregnant
- We were not going to choose IUI or IVF

Adoption discernment is hard and weird. Although God ultimately plans your family, it is not through selecting specific days for intercourse and letting nature run its course. There are many more decisions to make, involving the consideration of multiple factors, many unknowns, *and* multiple opportunities to *change your mind* along the way. This last part is something that many people don't understand and have no reason to unless they have been through it or know someone who has.

Once you begin the process, it's not like you sign your name in blood on the dotted line declaring that you must take home a certain child immediately. It is a slow process for which God has ample time to prepare your hearts for the right person. If you go through an agency, and hopefully find a good one, the social worker is a professional who does a lot of the hard work behind the scenes to make the proper connections in hopes of sparing both birth and adoptive families unnecessary stress and heartache. When an opportunity or opportunities to parent a child is/are presented, prospective adoptive parents can decline until the moment is right with no fear of judgement. It happens all the time. Chris and I declined to move forward with several potential birth mothers and babies before Bella was brought to our attention. It was freeing to learn that we had some control over something, and I think this fact will ease many hearts who are trying to determine if this is the right path for them.

Although there are certainly many components of adoption to consider, a really good starting place for this process of discernment is to spend time in prayer, together and separately, with these questions: "Are we called to be parents?" If the answer is yes, "Are we called to be parents right now or soon?"

After taking all the time we needed, we got two "yeses." So, we did some research, talked to friends with experience, and began filling out mounds of paperwork. Then it was time to wait––and trust. Then trust some more. Nothing suddenly became *easy* because we made this choice. God was still moving my heart into the right place. I knew this was the right next step for us, but I still struggled. The concept of adoption is natural for some people to wrap their heads around. I was *not* one of those people. It wasn't a topic of conversation in my home, in my church, or at my school. The only time I remember hearing anything about it was on TV–– and not in a positive light. Like it does for many others, it felt foreign to me. I had no real-life experience with adoption to round out the pointy edges of my perceptions, yet I knew I was called to mother a child.

Here is the important thing to remember––it's okay to feel that way. It is natural for anyone to have fears about bringing a child into their home. We don't *just* grow up expecting to have children, but also imagining whose eyes and whose mouth he or she will have. We are more likely to witness biological family connections than adoptive ones. It is hard to shake that uneasiness of wondering whether or not a child you don't personally conceive can *feel* fully your own rather than a bit foreign. But even with my concerns, God worked to open my heart to what seemed to me like an unusual and awkward situation, aligning not only my choice with his, but my desires as well. And as time passed, I grew more and more excited in anticipation of *finally* becoming a mom and meeting our baby girl regardless of the circumstances that would bring her to us. Marriage, parenthood–heck womanhood!–was looking nothing like what I expected for my future, but that didn't make it any less beautiful. It was actually becoming quite exhilarating.

About one year after starting the process, we were matched. Our social worker told us about a young woman who was pregnant with a little girl and due in a couple of months. There were a couple of things in our paperwork that didn't match this particular situation, like a higher financial commitment, but she shared it with us anyway.

We had already said no to two or three other opportunities that weren't right, but as we continued to chew on this one, we began to believe that something about it was different.

Thorough discernment took place over the next three days as we headed to Disneyworld for a trip Chris's parents bought for all their kids as a Christmas present and that we had planned several months prior. There was a clear conviction echoing throughout my heart that I repetitively shared with Chris: "Our daughter is our daughter no matter the cost." We pulled into the lot of our hotel after leaving the airport, put the car into park, looked at each other, and both confidently expressed that this was our daughter. We didn't wait another minute before giving our social worker the green light to connect us with her birth mother, in hopes that she would feel the same way. We called her before we even got out of the car.

A few days later, we were walking around Animal Kingdom–on what turned out to be a babymoon–when we got the news that she had chosen us. Time stopped for the second time in my life, but this time with good reason. We rejoiced like those crazy people you see in public and have no idea why they're hugging and high fiving. Maybe this really is the happiest place on earth? We snapped a picture on a bridge overlooking my favorite ride, *Mount Everest*, the exact spot where we learned of the news, and went back to that identical spot two and a half years later to take the same photo with our baby girl. There were two months to prepare for her arrival, and the several unexpected wrenches thrown into our plans during that time were no match for our newfound joy.

Her Birth Mother
Preparing for the special day that would officially make us parents consisted of both negative and positive plot twists. Getting to know Bella's birth mom was one of the positive ones. I'm embarrassed to admit that I went into the adoption process with a sense of ownership over our future child, even as she grew in the womb of another woman. I had an unfounded fear of her birth mom and the potential relationship she might insist on having with her child. Ultimately, it is rightly ordered for a birth mother to desire a healthy relationship with her child! This is a very good thing. But I want to be honest about my feelings and the process, a learning one filled with so many unknowns, and one that was scary on many levels. Even so, the woman who grew our baby girl became even more brave and even more of a hero to me with each encounter.

She is an immigrant who had been in the US for only three years, relocating from living with family in another state, mothering a one year old and three year old. She shared that she believed she could care for the two children she had, but not a third, and desired for her to have a better childhood than she had. She also expressed that she wanted to help a couple who couldn't have children. She spoke no English and had to rely solely on the only people she knew nearby–her new acquaintances at the adoption agency–for everything. Still, she boldly sacrificed her personal comforts and relationships to choose life and love for the new life growing inside of her. The world takes a quick look at a woman like her and sees weakness, but she was actually a resilient example of strength and selflessness.

It is interesting to think about the entirely different perspectives of the two women, one blessed with a pregnancy, however unplanned, and another blessed with an opportunity to raise that child, coming together for the same goal––to selflessly love another human. I will never forget the first time I laid eyes on Bella's birth mother. We walked around the corner of the apartment complex she was temporarily living in and knocked on the white door. Nervously awaiting the door to open like on a first date, I wondered what it would be like to meet our daughter's mother. I wanted her to like us. I wanted her to understand her incredible worth which was independent of this gift of parenthood she promised us. I wanted her to know how brave she was. And as that vertical separation gave way to the inside of her living room, I met eyes with a jet black-haired and dark-skinned petite young woman draped in tan and black leopard print, cautiously smiling. The language barrier meant we would have to work extra hard to communicate.

Would we meet her expectations? Would she be able to trust us with the life of her little girl? Would we be able to love her little girl as our own? These were all fair questions that I imagined were residing within the heart of the woman getting to know the two people who would become her daughter's parents.

And two very different but equally valued people who could mainly communicate through body language got to know each other slowly over the next couple of months. We played with her children, took her to the grocery, doctor appointments, and got to be present during an ultrasound. We took her to get her first pedicure and took her children to the park, investing quality time with them. We took her to lunch several times and learned that her favorite food is chicken wings. Her kids loved the "Despicable Me" movie, so we bought them the DVD and a portable player they could watch it on––while continuously mimicking the minions saying "buh-nah-nuh!" Fortunately, laughter, and love of minions, is universal.

I could not have anticipated how much our experience with this woman and her children would teach me. We experienced a world very different than the one we were used to and learned a lot from it. Meeting and caring for our daughter, a beautiful combination of her birth family and us, was expectedly life-changing in and of itself. I never imagined that the experience of her birth mother would be life-changing as well.

That strong woman labored by herself in her apartment for nearly a day before alerting the agency and heading to the hospital. We arrived about three hours after she gave birth to Bella, who was being lovingly clutched in her arms. There is something very important to take away from this story about birth mothers. When they choose to place their child for adoption, it is by no means a "giving up," nor is it any display of weakness, selfishness, or irresponsibility. It is an intentional and very difficult choice made out of unconditional love and pure strength!

It was equally as beautiful as it was painful to witness that moment in which she was clearly saying her goodbyes. The memory alone breaks my heart. It was an incredible visual of love in action unfolding in all of its perfection that I will treasure forever. I captured that moment with a photo that we can share with Bella who will hopefully always know how fervently she is loved by both of her mothers.

We gave her birth mother all the time she needed as we waited rather awkwardly in two chairs at the foot of her hospital bed. Eventually, the nurse walked over and asked her permission to bring Bella to us. With tears flowing freely down her cheeks and soaking into the bed sheets, she carefully handed the baby to the nurse, who handed her to me, who I handed to her daddy so I could go and comfort my hero. I needed her to know that she was not alone. I need her to know that we were not done with her because she has now entrusted us with her beloved child. I needed her to know how brave she was. I touched her arm and said, "You are a gift", as she drifted off to sleep, finally able to rest her exhausted eyes. And then I got to meet my daughter.

An Important Distinction
It is, admittedly, pretty easy for me to get all wide eyed and goofy-grinned when I talk about adoption because it gave us our daughter, and that would be enough! But it also expanded our understanding of love and gave us a much better perspective of women in crisis pregnancies and I am better because of it. But Chris and I aren't the only travelers on this journey, and the experiences for our other two travel companions, Bella and her birth mother, are each quite unique.

If I'm being brutally honest (again), prior to our adoption experience, I didn't really think of women with unplanned pregnancies with any depth. I had compassion for them on a superficial level and believed they have a responsibility to choose adoption over abortion if they choose not to parent, but without connecting that experience to the woman as a human person.

As someone who got a front row seat to the process, I can't imagine a situation that would ever be as simple or easy as "just giving your child up for adoption." We need to remove that sentence from our vocabulary!

What I encountered in Bella's birth mother was a human being who was scared, alone, and both fully aware of and in love with the human she was carrying, willing to give up great amounts of emotional and physical comforts for the sake of her baby. Clearly, every birth mom is unique. But can you fathom a situation in which parting with your own flesh and blood would not be incredibly confusing and difficult considering the innate biological connection between mother and child? It is nothing short of traumatic.

I witnessed the painful clutches of a birth mother's love. The decision to place her child for adoption was an enormous act of love that did not come without great sacrifice! She deserves to be respected, not oversimplified. In a perfect world, she'd be able to raise her daughter within a committed marriage and with appropriate support. We'd be able to get pregnant. We do not live in a perfect world, but God has conquered death! He is the God of the living (Luke 20: 37-38) and He used two imperfect situations to provide a loving home for an unexpected child––the sole reason why two families who probably would have never united, come together.

As much as I've talked about myself and Bella's birth mother, adoption doesn't exist for us. It exists solely for the sake of the child. It is, or should be, void of self. It wills the good of another; two great acts of love. And although Bella is happy and being raised in a loving home surrounded by a big family and lots of friends who care deeply for her, she carries an unknown trauma with her as well. Her realization of this wound will evolve over time, and none of that is lost on us as adoptive parents.

Adoption itself is never a perfect scenario. And unfortunately, some adoption situations add unnecessary trauma. But many adoptions add a lot of good to an imperfect situation. Chris and I can't take that pain and confusion away, but we can create an atmosphere where her curiosity is encouraged, where she feels the freedom to question and explore her origins, and feel however she feels without judgement––even when some of it is hard for us to hear.

Our role is to support her when she feels that loss, to support her desire to discover her roots at her pace, and to provide the loving home that we promised her birth mother we would give her. That means loving her right where she is–– whether she's feeling the joy of our family, missing the one that's farther away, or a little of both. It will be a lifelong learning experience for all of us.

Even within the imperfect situation, I'll tell you a few things. Our girl knows joy. She knows she is loved. You can love more than one family with your whole heart. We cannot fully understand adoption until we integrate the three pieces of this complex puzzle–adoptive parents, birth family, and child–realizing that the joy of bringing the child into a loving home does not come without the great growing pains of sacrificial love.

Parents at Last

I hope that sharing my perspective of birth mothers and our adopted daughter gives some valuable insight into a world many don't see, but it is limited to what I have perceived from the outside. My personal experience as an adoptive mother allows me to provide much more depth because I have lived it and understand the concerns firsthand. There are many infertile women called to adopt, but are paralyzed, like me, by fear and confusion as to what that means and what it will be like. Like each birth mother, each adoptive mother is unique, but this adoptive mother felt every worry melt away without effort even before embracing our new daughter for the first time.

On the day of Bella's birth, I was able to witness one of my *new* dreams coming true and felt zero regret about not welcoming our first child through pregnancy. Our experience was special and memorable just like with every mother who gives birth. We continued to pray for Bella's birth mom as we effortlessly dove into parenthood. The concerns I had faded into the background like a distant dream as Chris and I both experienced nothing but pure joy; our hearts soaring for months.

The verdict on whether or not she would *feel* like ours was in well before Bella was born. The moment we learned that her "tummy mommy" chose us, we began to *feel* like her parents. Adoption is not about whether or not that child will ever feel like your own, but about whether or not it is what God is calling you to. My fears about biology were just that––fears. And fear has nothing to do with discernment. Once Bella was put into our arms, there was absolutely no difference between our reality as adoptive parents and what we anticipated as parents of a biological child. It was also a blessing to be fully rested and not have to recover physically.

The only thing I miss *to this day* is the inability to feel new life growing inside of me. That is a pain I will always have, but pregnancies come and go. God willing, we will have our daughter for much longer than a gestation period. Some family members are grown from within and some are welcomed in from outside. Our plans were far surpassed by what God designed especially for us, and that has taken some of the sting out of infertility. He has not forgotten us, but set aside a unique child (or children) *for us*, just as he does for every couple blessed with pregnancies.

Cost
Let's not pretend that adoption doesn't come with plenty of strings and footnotes attached. The reality is that we were very fortunate to have the means to adopt and to have our first attempt be successful. There are many couples who experience the deep pain of failed adoption(s), which is an experience I cannot imagine or relate to. Many don't even attempt because it is so expensive. Even when successful, the process from start to finish carries many stressors and frustrations. We became familiar with many of these throughout this learn-as-you-go operation.

It begins with mounds of paperwork and several home studies, all of which felt pretty invasive. It makes perfect sense that people must prove they aren't criminals and have the correct motivations to adopt a child, but that doesn't make you *feel* any more comfortable about others poking and prodding through your entire life. We were required to have FBI background checks, get fingerprinted, get reference letters from four different friends and two different family members who could vouch for us as decent human beings, and even "prove" my infertility. That last one especially felt like a punch to the gut.

We didn't research agencies (mistake #1). Friends of Chris and I were pleased with a lawyer and social worker they used, so we moved forward with that recommendation. However, the birth mother to their daughter didn't contact the agency to find adoptive parents until the baby was born, so their experience directly with the agency was minimal. They only knew the faces of the lawyer and social worker, whom we could all agree were splendid to work with. We were selected by a birth mother who resided about three hours away from us, near the agency she connected with. With approximately two months until her due date and the agency directly caring for her, we were required to get acquainted with our middleman whom we found to be unprofessional, delayed in providing important information, and okay with cutting corners. Despite these troubles, this was the route it took to meet our baby girl, and we are grateful for that.

In addition to agency drama, there is an underlying fear that the birth mother will change her mind. In Louisiana, the woman *must* wait three days after giving birth to sign over her rights, a point by which our hearts had already been fully invested. Needless to say, it was scary, but God thankfully provided the grace we needed to get through it. Financial risk varies depending on the agency chosen, but there is always a possibility to lose money already spent in caring for her and any children she may have before she even gives birth. There is also a risk for the birth father to suddenly appear and take an interest in the baby.

Even after Bella's birth mother signed over her rights, we were required to hire a private investigator through our agency to try and find her birth father and request that he sign over his rights. If he decided that he wanted to raise the baby, he would have had to prove that he provided for her birth mother while pregnant, but he could've taken us to court to try.

If he does nothing or is not found after six months, a judge will hopefully finalize the adoption. Bella's birth father made no attempts.

There are also other uncomfortable realities to consider. Every single adoption experience is unique because every person and situation is unique. There are no guarantees; only ample opportunities to trust in God as you venture deeper and deeper into the unknown with a growing understanding that no child belongs to any human—all belong to God. Adoption is not a cure for infertility, a promise of a smooth transition into parenthood, or a "back-up" plan. It is not second best to pregnancy or a consolation prize. It is either meant for a family, with or without biological kids, or it is not. God did not promise me a life without challenges, but he did promise that he would never leave or forsake me. He has more than "earned" my trust despite the appearance of my life, and the struggles included, to the outside world.

But please do consider these aspects of adoption before ever simply offering advice such as, "you can always *just* adopt," as if it's an easy and straightforward replacement for pregnancy. That is far from the truth and can cause great discomfort and frustration within the heart of the infertile. Also reconsider sharing thoughts like, "many people start the adoption process and then get pregnant." It dismisses the pain of the couple and often makes them feel personally accountable for their inability to get pregnant.

If It's Good for Him, It's Good for Us

As I write this, I am rummaging through old memories trying to remember that feeling of concern about having a child that is not biological. I remember not being able to grasp the idea of equality between biology and adoption. It isn't something I ever said out loud, but I believed internally that one was superior to the other. Then I step back into my present reality and it disproves that concept with no effort at all. Bella is no less a part of our family than any other member would have been. And although we didn't *make* her in the traditional sense, we have formed her in ways that no other two people could have. And she has done the same for us.

Having this knowledge and experience, which I understand not everyone is privileged to, leads to more questions and skepticism about IUI and IVF with all of its expenses and low effectiveness rates. How is it worth it? How can we think we will only be satisfied by having a biological child through these means? How much would we have missed out on had we tried artificial reproductive technologies? Do we know how good God is? Our daughter is perfectly ours the way she is. How many children don't biologically resemble their parents at all? How many parents don't choose to love their own biological children? God has claimed *us* as his own adopted sons and daughters! We hear it at Mass on the feast of the Holy Family: "God our Father, we your adopted sons and daughters offer these prayers as members of your holy family..." Look at what scripture says about adoption: "*...In love, he destined us for adoption to himself through Jesus Christ, in accord with the favor of his will, [6] for the praise of the glory of his grace that he granted us in the beloved.*"
-Ephesians 1:4-6 (NABRE)

"*God sent his Son, born of a woman, born under the law, [5] to ransom those under the law, so that we might receive adoption. [6] As proof that you are children,[a] God sent the spirit of his Son into our hearts, crying out, "Abba, Father!" [7] So you are no longer a slave but a child, and if a child then also an heir, through God.*"
-Galatians 4:4-7 (NABRE)

"*⁷ ...nor are they all children of Abraham because they are his descendants; but "It is through Isaac that descendants shall bear your name." ⁸ This means that it is not the children of the flesh who are the children of God, but the children of the promise are counted as descendants.*"
-Romans 9:7-8 (NABRE)

"*¹² But to those who did accept him he gave power to become children of God, to those who believe in his name, ¹³ [b]who were born not by natural generation nor by human choice nor by a man's decision but of God*"
.-John 1:12-13 (NABRE)

"*¹ [a]See what love the Father has bestowed on us that we may be called the children of God. Yet so we are. The reason the world does not know us is that it did not know him. ² Beloved, we are God's children now...*"
-1 John 3:1-2 (NABRE)

"*²⁶ For through faith you are all children of God[a] in Christ Jesus.*"
-Galatians 3:26 (NABRE)

These are a few of over sixty other verses I found in Scripture. And what a privilege it is to be a daughter and son of God, Himself, in all of His glory! If adoption is good enough for Him, then it is more than good enough for us.

Funny Thing Is...
God doesn't always answer our prayers in the way we anticipate, but he always exceeds our expectations when we let Him. He won't impose His will on us because He respects our freedom to make choices, but He never

disappoints when we let him take control. Adoption is not part of every infertile person's call to holiness, but *something* is.

We immediately embraced Bella as our own, and as soon as her personality began to develop, both friends and strangers began to marvel at how much she actually *does* resemble us—specifically in the way her smile and other facial expressions, and the way she talks, match both mine and my husband's. Chris's sister, Kim, recently told me that she even stands like me. She also told us that she cannot imagine our family without her, adding, "Isn't it funny how things work out?" It continues to both baffle me and hug my heart every time the words "she looks just like you" hit our ears.

It is the combination of all of her features and both of her cultures—hair color, stature, likes and dislikes, accent (or lack thereof), facial expressions and more that make her who she is: a tangible form of God's love for us, blessing us with her presence each day. Although she doesn't fully understand everything yet, she already knows her "tummy mommy" by name and is able to see herself being embraced by her as a newborn in a picture in her bedroom. She prays for her and her half siblings by name every night. She can even explain that her birth mother allowed mommy and daddy to raise her because she loves her so much.

In the previous chapter, I discussed the gifts God has designed for our lives. My gifts only truly began to blossom because of how I chose, with God's grace, to live through my suffering and infertility. But what is paramount to me is that Bella would have been enough. Had I *not* begun my incredibly fulfilling and fruitful ministry, public speaking, writing, and rapping, my life would be *full* by raising our adopted daughter Bella, alone. But God is *so* generous and he cannot be outdone. He continues to share himself by lavishly adorning us with more and more.

Yes, he is that good. Yes, you are worth it. When we give Him our trust, He rewards us with immeasurable satisfaction.

CHAPTER 10

ViCTRiX

"You may not realize it when it happens, but a kick in the teeth may be the best thing in the world for you."
— Walt Disney

THE LIGHTS WERE DIMMED LOW and the darkness was pierced only by flashing neon lights and cell phones ready to record the show. The atmosphere of a concert was set. The bass danced out of the speakers and vibrated onto my skin. Over one hundred teens approached the stage with their hands raised and knees bouncing along with the beat, ready to be entertained. The adults followed suit behind them. My heart pounded with each passing second as I waited for my name to be called by the headliner on stage. I was about to join him for my very first rap performance.

I can imagine the look of confusion that I have just painted across your face.

God can make some pretty remarkable things happen when given some trust, but I could've never dreamed up some of the things He would invite me to explore. Rapping is one of those things. If you ask me to put some music on, nine times out of ten it's going to include some bass and a good beat. It's definitely not everyone's favorite kind of music, but it's hard to deny the artistry required to match meaningful lyrics/rhymes with catchy sounds. In high school (Uptown New Orleans), we warmed up for basketball games to the cleanest versions we could find of select hip-hop tunes. Part of our "free throw celebration" was Juvenile's *Nolia Clap* (do yourself a favor and *don't* look it up).

One of my besties and I jammed our way to and from school daily to our mixed CDs (remember those?) of Nelly, Cash Money Millionaires, Eminem, Ying Yang Twins, 50 Cent, and much more. I know––those weren't the best role models to help shape us as young women who understand our worth *and* basic human dignity. But those were the types of beats that reached into my soul and moved it.

Eminem is one of the world's most famous rappers. His first song was superficial and straight up dirty, but it broadcasted his incredible skill. If you kept up, he would eventually combine his intense pain from some incredibly difficult life experiences with his *gift* of lyricism to produce some of the most impressive rap music that exists. Like it or not–tasteful or not–you can't deny his skill. He is revered by many as the greatest rapper of all time. Take away the vulgarity and his ability to express his emotions creatively is something I really respect and connect with.

Many associate rapping with vulgarity, but it *is* possible to glorify God and uplift people through music by choosing the right words after handing the pen to the Holy Spirit. I didn't know this until recently, but there are many rappers who are gifted at delivering their message with positivity and in light of Christian values. Some of my personal favorites are NF, Lecrae, Andy Mineo, and Oscar "TwoTen" Rivera. This may not be your typical kind of evangelization, but that doesn't make it any less impactful as a means to draw the hearts of those who connect with this kind of music closer to the heart of Christ.

When thinking about God, love and mercy are probably the first couple of things that come to mind. One aspect of God that few describe, but consistently fascinates me, is His creativity. We see it displayed in a variety of ways in the arts: paint and graphite strokes of genius, sculpturing, humor, combining emotion and imagination for moving pictures, and expressing emotion through rhyme, rhythms, and spoken word. The most amazing talents we witness in the world, both usual and unusual, have come straight from God's fingertips and vary, with the purpose of relating to us individually. We can choose to use our own gifts for good and sometimes that requires thinking outside of the box.

I knew this style of music moved me, but I never considered myself musical. I've never played an instrument and have a singing voice that could kill a cat. The only reason I first attempted to put words to music was because Chris and I wanted to do something unique for our first dance as husband and wife. Rapping, of course, was at the top of the list and I had no idea if we could pull it off, but we did. It turns out that nothing confuses and pleasantly surprises your guests more than a good old-fashioned *wedding rap*. I will never forget lying in my bed one night and opening myself up to the ability of writing lyrics. As I searched my brain for words, they began to string themselves together without effort. I turned over, grabbed my phone, and typed in most of my first song into the "notes" app.

It wasn't the most incredible thing I'd ever write, but it was creative *enough* to give us and our wedding guests a thrill. The first verse ends with:

Beautiful party, tuxes and dresses
We couldn't be happier if we drove off in a Lexus
Best family and friends two people could ask for
If ya holla at me–you better get on the dance floor...

I would do most of the rapping, but I couldn't leave my new husband out. When he's not listening to Country music, Chris will throw on some music we can bounce to and jam with me. But like most people, he has never had a desire to rap anything in his life. Still, he needed a part in our song. He *sort of* nailed it, but let's just say that he's going to stick to his career mastering oil and gas engineering. Here is the small part I wrote for him:

This just in–your favorite combination to appear
A PTA/rapper and an electrical engineer.

The song goes on:

We step out these doors and start our life together
God gave us a bond that's thicker than leather
You can call me Mrs. Chris!
Even Mr. Cutco couldn't sever this...

You've got me crazy, speaking Spanish like tres, dos, uno
And soaring on a rocket to Mars, like Bruno
Bruno, Bruno, That's my new name, oh!
Martin, don't you worry 'cuz this lion's been tamed, oh!

Our bridal party had no idea we were about to light up the reception hall with a mini rap concert after our first dance. They were thrilled to surround us during the performance like revered groupies and still comment on the CD we burned and distributed as favors to this day. I loved being a newlywed. And at the time, my perfectly planned life sequence had not yet hit its hiccup because we saved sex for marriage, making us unaware of our infertility.

We were a legit stereotypical newly-married Catholic couple. I really enjoyed flexing my anatomy and physiology muscles and helping others as a physical therapist assistant. We received the Sacraments, hung out with friends and family, participated in a few private prayer groups, did some traveling, and really enjoyed life while waiting for pregnancy to *just happen*. We had great experiences, but I was unaware that I wasn't pushing my creativity and diving into *all* of my God-given talents.

Outlet
A little over one year into marriage, my physical pain began to increase and my fourth and fifth surgeries were scheduled. This was the first time the terrifying words "adenomyosis" and "hysterectomy" were mentioned to me, officially starting the countdown to what felt like a ticking time bomb of my fertility. Getting pregnant at this point was not an option, but something that I *just needed to happen*, especially now that I felt the pressure of the clock. I'm not suggesting that that was a healthy disposition to have, just describing reality. Between the severe physical symptoms and my very real fears, I needed to share this struggle with the world. I needed to find *my* outlet, and that is when I wrote my very first blog.

That, too, was far from my best work. But it got my creative juices flowing and it felt amazing to express my emotions in this way. As I continued to write, I found that I *loved* to play around with all kinds of imagery by using words to paint authentic pictures of real life experiences––no matter how ugly. If you follow my writing over the years, you'll notice a trend of joy through sorrow, from deep pain to acceptance, and a slight tone of bitterness that slowly improved as that acceptance became more concrete. I had been bitten by the writing bug and I thank God for it because it has been incredibly cathartic not only for me, but for others who suffer and haven't yet found their voice to share about it.

I just laughed out loud as I re-read "slight tone of bitterness." I worked hard to conceal this in my writing, but in reality, it was more of an obvious and outright cynical tone of bitterness. Before I was able to distance myself from fertile women and clear my head of comparisons, I dealt with my pain by poking fun at myself and exaggerating my perceptions of them. I eventually came up with what I considered to be some hilarious punch lines.

I thought, "This stuff is too good. What can I do with it?" It was actually perfect for a stand-up comedy routine. Most of the material *was* inspired by real life situations. But that thought appealed to me for less time than it took for me to get the words out of my mouth. Then a light bulb turned on as I realized I wrote that *wedding rap* a year or so prior. I can still remember that "ah-ha" moment when one of my eyebrows arched up as if to carry a most intriguing idea. And that was when "There's No Baby in this King Cake," my next song, and first of full length, began to take shape:

Another month down–can't get it right
Only thing late about mine is when it starts at midnight!
I wonder what it's like to be a "normal couple?"
Your man looks at your stuff and you get knocked up.
I don't count down weeks or squeeze tiny cheeks...
My husband looks at me and I know–

I'm about to get a visit from my CRAZY Aunt Flow.
I get cramps and aches from my head to my toes–
I've got that waddle walk down, but no baby to show!
They've got special parking for mothers expecting–
I need a spot too! ...when my body's rejecting–
The inner lining of my uterus is falling
Another negative test sends me balling...

Hook:
We want a baby of our own
To raise til he's grown
Feel like a chord without a phone–
Disconnected; no dial tone
My hubby likes me a lot, givin' kisses by the dozen
I got a whole lot of lovin' but no but in the oven

Final lines:
...Look closely you'll see the test was no mistake
There's no baby in this king cake
Just you and me livin' life by the lake
There's no baby in this king cake

This title and closing lyric was inspired by a real life event. You know I grew up and got married near and in New Orleans, Louisiana, where we are known for our cinnamon and sugary tastes of heaven with babies stuffed inside. Meet the "King Cake." The tradition calls for whoever finds the baby to buy the next one. One Mardi Gras season, Chris and I finished up a king cake in our kitchen and realized that neither of us ever got the baby. They had actually forgotten to put one in our box!

After I busted out in obnoxious laughter, the room turned cold. I was hit with a bitter realization of our situation and felt the emphasis of feeling forgotten myself. As you read those lyrics, you were probably either moderately entertained or felt sorry for the person who wrote them, or a little of both. I have mixed feelings about it myself, but nevertheless, it is real life. While the whole song is catchy and clever, it presents a painfully realistic snapshot of what goes on inside the mind of the average infertile woman at some point in their journey––and begs for someone to hear her heart cry.

Battle Wounds
Several months after those two additional surgeries and about two years after we got married brought on my "worst day ever." As described previously, it dropped me to rock bottom, but only to re-align my focus and center my heart on my Creator who would give me everything I need in life, and then some. That day and those that followed, which were sprinkled with my new companionship with St. Teresa of Avila, rejuvenated me. Of course, I needed to write! I wrote plenty of blogs, but there was a tug on my heart to express myself creatively in a different way; one that allowed me to physically emote an honest story of hope in the midst of deep pain and mourning––and this time, with more vulnerability.

At this point, I had had six surgeries giving me ten unique scars, which resemble stripes of varying lengths, all around my belly. By the time the song was recorded, I'd had eleven surgeries. As I changed my clothes daily and hopped in the shower, I would notice the uneven marks and rough patches on my skin, but I wasn't ashamed. Those scars cut deep, both literally and figuratively, signifying so much of what I have been through and overcome. I was proud to tell the story of these wounds, which represent the physical, emotional, and spiritual battles that I have fought and won despite the suffering, and despite the absence of that one thing I so desperately wanted.

I was excited to have the opportunity to connect words with experiences and emotions that so many women feel and don't know how to express. All of this gave *birth* to my first "real" rap song. "Battle Wounds" was intentionally written as a reflection of my specific battles with pain and infertility, but in a way that anyone can relate to, regardless of the details.

Verse 1:
I never said "Yes" to this trouble or that
Don't drive over spikes and get surprised by a flat!
But the jabs keep comin'– every month gettin' harder
I'd put up my shield, but they don't make armor
Count em–ten stripes deep; they've made me who I am
Eleven laps on this track, but I still stand!
Ignorant of reality and blinded by fear

I started on this journey and it became my career
Tempted to hide and let my jealous flag fly
To live on the edge and let bitterness rise
I've got to focus on the most of the good in life
Commit or bust–He turned my fuss into trust
The pain lives on, but my faith runs deep
Don't give up now 'cuz victory ain't cheap!
Perpendicular boards bringin' my only relief!
Don't give up now, 'cuz victory ain't cheap.

Hook:
I'm stuck on this coaster and I can't get off
My wheels are rusted' over, but I can't get off
My knuckles turnin' white from holdin' on so hard
I better let go now and embrace these scars...

This song gave me such strength! I would use the words as some sort of anthem to motivate me to get through the moments when I suffered most, physically and emotionally. I felt like God had written some pretty interesting and soul-touching poetry through my hands and I wanted to share it with others, but I had zero confidence in my abilities. Rapping? Are you serious? What kind of olive-skinned Catholic girl do I think I am? I assumed no one would take me seriously and was embarrassed to put my lyricism on display for even my closest friends. So, I did what any normal insecure twenty-something year old would do-- I emailed it to myself to remain hidden for the next couple of years.

Rapping definitely fell into Jen Fulwiler's "Your Blue Flame[17]" concept, specifically from Chapter 8: "You Can Finally Accept Yourself." Fulwiler makes an excellent connection between shame and insecurity.

"We need to watch out for this because one of the main ways we miss discovering our blue flames is by smothering them in shame. Shame is a great hiding place for our insecurities. It's often a Trojan horse that lets an army of fears invade and hold us hostage."

Fulwiler goes on to joke about what some people would consider crazy about Marie Kondo's blue flame. And I certainly thought I was crazy.

"This is not normal! Some people may have even thought she had a psychological disorder. Many people with such an unusual personality would squelch their natural tendencies in fear of seeming strange. Thank goodness Marie didn't. She embraced her quirks and started a home-organizing business, eventually writing wildly popular books that turned into a hit Netflix show. By embracing her unique way of seeing the world, she has helped millions of people take control of their lives and their spaces. The rest of us would do well to take a page from her bold acceptance of her own eccentricities…"

Although I'm no hit Netflix show, I can absolutely identify with that way of thinking. It actually *wasn't* the right time to share that side of myself, but I didn't have the awareness to recognize the difference between choosing to wait as I honed my new craft and hiding it out of shame. I had a lot of work to do internally to allow the person God was molding me into to take shape.

In the meantime, we started the adoption process, I quit my job as a PTA as we welcomed Bella into our home, and I became a core team member for a local youth group as I witnessed one of my best friends, Elise, grab hold of her life-long dream to become a Youth Director at a supportive parish. Our friendship spans over a decade, during a time of which we have experienced a long and colorful list of joys and heartbreaks together. Oh yea, and she is infertile, too! Our relationship is deep, fostering continued growth in spirituality with a healthy dose of accountability. In short, she makes me a better person.

When she was hanging out at my house one day, I felt a strange and random tug from the Holy Spirit to dig through my emails to find and show her my "Battle Wounds" lyrics that had been safely hidden and stored under lock and key. I mustered up the courage to hand her the three verses and one hook displayed on my phone, then sat back and prepared myself for an obligatory pat on the back followed by a "nice effort, kiddo."

But that didn't happen.

I watched her eyebrows slowly rise and her jaw inch slowly towards the floor. Even she was surprised at how captivated she was by the written words. I wasn't lying when I said we hold each other accountable––Elise is always painfully honest with me, and she isn't easily impressed when it comes to creativity. My lyrics actually moved her. When she finished reading the song, the way she looked at and spoke to me affirmed and encouraged me in a way I didn't know I needed. That was the day a little spark ignited inside of me, and ViCTRiX was born.

Female Victor
ViCTRiX, the rap name Elise later helped me to create, is Latin for "female victor." Latin is the language of the Church Christ instituted, and that I hold so closely to my heart. A "victor" is "a person who has overcome or defeated an adversary; a conqueror (Dictionary.com)." I hope ViCTRiX communicates the hope and joy that is possible through great trials, even when the end result is not what was planned for. We all battle daily and victory doesn't always come in the ways we expect.

The timing of that tug to "come out" as a female rapper to my friend could not have been more perfect. Elise and her husband had planned the most impressive local retreat I have ever experienced. They invited some well-known speakers, hired an established band, equipped the room with professional audio and visual components, set the ambiance, provided numerous priests for confession, a well-formed junior core team, and flew in an old friend from Franciscan University of Steubenville and now International speaker, emcee, and rapper, Oscar "TwoTen" Rivera, to give a talk and perform at a lunch-time concert on Saturday.

I was excited. I had been entertained by one Catholic/Christian rapper at one or two Steubenville conferences many years ago (Do y'all remember Bob Lefnesky/Righteous B?), but other than that, I was unaware that it was actually a *thing* anyone was doing well at the time. I was eager to hear this guy out, and maybe even meet him.

On the morning of the concert, I just happened to pass Oscar in the main hall and I was shocked as he kindly spoke words to me (I am shy and generally/never initiate convos with strangers or even non-strangers), expressing that his wife was a fan of me because of my *Taking Back the Terms* (now @whitelotusblooming and @fabmbase) outreach.

My newfound and growing confidence was responsible for making the following words come out of my mouth: "Really?! Thank you! I am a fan of yours. (Wait for it....) I'm a rapper, too!"

What? Did I really just refer to myself as a rapper because I dug up one song I wrote years ago? And to someone who actually *is* a rapper?

I can only imagine what was running through his mind as I chewed on the not-so-tasty fact that I could not put the words back into my mouth and as he stared at someone who looks like me and just referred to herself as a rapper. But to my complete amazement, the words did not make him run away, but intrigued and even excited him a little bit.

He said: "Really? Do. You. Want. To. Do. Something. With. Me. On. Stage?" (He didn't stop after each word. I just heard it in slow motion.) My heart pounded. The spark grew. And as I shared the second verse of "Battle Wounds" with him to prepare for our performance, he, too; a stranger experienced in his field, affirmed me, and watered the seeds of passion and talent God planted inside of me so that I could finally sprinkle it into the world.

We performed for well over one hundred teens that day under the flashing neon lights and formed a collaboration team and friendship that continues to grow today. Then we did it all over again for that same retreat the next year, but this time with a brand new song we wrote together, "*Holy Family,*" and one verse of a new song about the Eucharist I had written after that first retreat using the beat from Lil Wayne's "A Milli." It was epic. I had been bitten by the writing bug again, but this time directed my passion towards lyrics to uplift hearts and point them towards God. I now have six songs written. The first song I recorded was an introduction to ViCTRiX & a collaboration I wrote with Oscar called "*Pen & the Beast*" after performing at that second retreat:

I'm a mommy by day and slayin' dragons by night
Got my voice as my sword and my faith is my bite
Y'all, I got into this game about two minutes ago
I was gripping tight to my pain and tryin' to let it go
My heart bleeds words begging to become lyrics

He said lean into the strange–you can't say "no" to the Spirit!
Tried to hold the monster back and keep her locked in her cage
But this beat is in my bones–put this monster on stage!
Gotta keep yourself in check and know the goal, gotta stay small
'Cuz the dark can't get enough, it's full of self, gonna be its own downfall
He needs to increase while I decrease if I'm gonna survive
'Cuz you know you gotta be counter-cultural, go against the stream, gonna get me eternal life!

I was captivated by the idea of rapping and the way the beats moved me when I was younger, yet I never once considered tapping into that desire until my experiences called for it. Even then, I questioned it because it seemed so unconventional. But who was I to judge God's creativity within me? I am finally able to accept this ability within myself regardless of what others may think about it. My music isn't well known and I don't think I'll be performing at the Grammys any time soon, but by engaging in one of the many things that makes me come alive, I am appreciating a gift God has so generously given to me—once again breathing new life into the world. The purpose of sharing our gifts is not to get recognition, but to use them no matter what anyone else thinks. It is about being honest with ourselves about who we are and how we were created. This is true humility.

There is another aspect of this story that also deserves some credit, and that's the power of friendship. Other people, whether they are friends, strangers, or acquaintances, impact our lives daily to varying degrees. This has been a tremendous blessing in my life, but also cause for great difficulty. So, I will give you a peek behind the curtain to the astounding influences others have had on my particular experience of suffering.

If you want to hear some of Mary's music, find the "Rapping" IGTV series in her bio on Instagram @WhiteLotusBlooming.

CHAPTER 11

Them

"What does love look like? It has the hands to help others. It has the feet to hasten to the poor and needy. It has eyes to see misery and want. It has the ears to hear the sighs and sorrows of men. That is what love looks like."
— Saint Augustine

BEING INFERTILE IN A SEA of fertile women is like being a house cat in the jungle. You can walk around like you own the place until the real wild cats show up, causing you to instantly put up your guard. You sense them from a mile away and instantly tense up. They won't smell your fear because you've learned to hide it well. You try to fit in, seeing as you *are* the same species, but you undoubtedly won't keep up. The cheetahs naturally talk about how fast they are. The tigers gravitate towards each other because they understand what it's like to be so incredibly strong. You know nothing about their speed and strength except that you have desperately yearned to experience it yourself. They try to teach you how to be like them, as if it were that simple. Every moment is another reminder of your insufficiencies. You pray they will see you–not just the fact that you're present in the same space, but to have the awareness of their actions *and* your pain–so as not to accidentally crush you.

I have conquered a lot. Becoming familiar with a level of acceptance that has largely diminished the steep drops of that monthly roller coaster is not without sadness, but it is freeing. And although I have received a lot of healing in this department, there is one dimension of this journey that I have and continue to struggle with most, and that's encountering fertile people *"in the wild."*

You can take a pregnancy test and emotionally prepare for disappointment in the privacy of your own home and choose to stay hidden during certain times that, for whatever reason, are particularly painful. But you can't always anticipate spotting that perfect baby bump when out and about, or that person who is unaware of how to talk sensitively about their own fertility. You can hardly relate to conversations about things you've never experienced. You can't beg someone to see your invisible pain. You can't always control your facial expression in response to yet another pregnancy announcement or gender reveal. And you can't punch a person in the face for giving you more unsolicited infertility advice.

I have already admitted that my bitterness was pretty strong for a long time and despite my best efforts, I am not sure how well I hid it or showed kindness when I was at my weakest. Figuring out how to navigate my apparent fertility status while surrounded by my closest girlfriends who are almost always bursting with the most adorable pregnant bellies and newborns has been challenging at best. They do nothing wrong by simply being fertile. But it soon began to feel incredibly depressing to merely exist in their presence. Pregnant women, especially of the Catholic variety, became warped in my mind and placed into an imaginary category of me vs. "them."

I remember one gathering at a friend's house where nine of those bellies were counted around me as they all smiled for a picture. Nine! At another event which happened to be a child's birthday party, I walked into the home and became so overwhelmed with all the children that I had to rush out to escape what I felt to be the walls closing in around me. During a Baptism, when the priest began pouring water over the baby's head, I suddenly became crushed with grief and was luckily able to sneak into the bathroom just before uncontrollably bursting into tears. The only blog I ever went back and deleted was entitled "Harsh Reality: Enter at Your Own Risk." I'll leave that one up to your imagination.

I had never experienced such public anxiety. I was surrounded by too many reminders of my insufficiencies to believe that I was enough, since I didn't match so many other Catholic women. This was another unintended side effect of growing up in a wonderful Catholic culture that appropriately supports new life and families, but often without the balance of welcoming those on the other end of the fertility spectrum and, again, the priceless gift of spiritual motherhood. Those who are infertile aren't the only ones to experience this. Spiritual parenthood is something that should penetrate all of our lives, lifting the marginalized. There is undoubtedly an essential **need** for **all** people in church regardless of sex, hair or skin color, and ability to do anything, procreation included. 1 Corinthians 12: 12-23 (NABRE) is one of my favorites, as we hear Paul describe that:

"[12] As a body is one though it has many parts, and all the parts of the body, though many, are one body, so also Christ. [13] For in one Spirit we were all baptized into one body...[14] Now the body is not a single part, but many. [15] If a foot should say, "Because I am not a hand I do not belong to the body," it does not for this reason belong any less to the body... [17] If the whole body were an eye, where would the hearing be?... [21] The eye cannot

say to the hand, "I do not need you..." [22] *Indeed, the parts of the body that seem to be weaker are all the more necessary,* [23] *and those parts of the body that we consider less honorable we surround with greater honor..."*

Verses 27-31 (NABRE) add an important point that accentuates the use of our gifts via spiritual parenthood.

"[27] Now you are Christ's body, and individually parts of it. [28] Some people God has designated in the church to be, first, apostles;[a] second, prophets; third, teachers; then, mighty deeds; then, gifts of healing, assistance, administration, and varieties of tongues. [29] Are all apostles? Are all prophets? Are all teachers? Do all work mighty deeds? [30] Do all have gifts of healing? Do all speak in tongues? Do all interpret? [31] Strive eagerly for the greatest spiritual gifts."

Notice that nowhere in Scripture does it simply encourage to eagerly desire a *greater* family size. Yet, silent judgements and accusations regarding contraception are frequently felt by many whose families don't line up with certain expectations. Women and men at both ends of the fertility spectrum often become victims of these drive-by prying eyes. Both jokes and complaints in mixed company about how easy it is to get pregnant are common at every gathering. Mother's Day Mass has become more than offering prayers and recognition of the feminine genius. It is often dreaded by the invisible infertile who are usually forced to watch as biological motherhood is hailed as a superior good. The acknowledgements in these Bible passages are inherent Catholic beliefs and teachings, but it is not always clearly communicated to us, allowing us to *feel* as connected and included as Christ intended.

Healthy Boundaries

So, I missed the message that I was an equally important human in the eyes of the Church despite my inability to have children. I lost sight of myself and sank into a deep depression. It wasn't just church people I struggled to be around. Pregnancies and new babies bring an incredible amount of joy and beauty into the world, but they also deliver many challenges. Both that joy and those challenges tend to be indiscriminately shouted from the rooftops––as they should be! However, it is often to the detriment of an unintended, or *unknown*, audience of women struggling with infertility. I *had* to create some separation from at least some of the things that were constantly poking at my pain so that I could find my place and begin to heal.

The hardest part about that was simply giving myself permission to set some healthy boundaries because my mental health *is* so important. *Mental and emotional health are essential dimensions of the human person!* We are always called to look for Christ in and be Christ to others, especially when it is hard, but we are not called to put ourselves in situations that are likely to cause us harm. For a long time, I forced myself to be present and fake niceties at the expense of my own sense of self-worth and health. I was unaware of it at the time, but that was not what God *or my friends* would have ever asked of me. I eventually tried to communicate my need for distance with respect and hope I was successful.

I politely asked friends to remove me from group text messages that often broke into chats about children, birthing, schooling, and pregnancies. I kept up with close friends in smaller private texts and still enjoyed the girls' nights. I explained as minimally as possible to each person who invited me/us to a children's birthday party, Baptism, or baby shower that we wouldn't make it and sent a gift when applicable. Eventually we would attend some of these events again, but we needed that distance initially. I still choose not to attend most baby showers. I grew closer to my only other infertile friends, which were few, and we grasped each other tightly as we both rode the roller coaster of infertility.

And you know what? Everyone understood—and probably learned a little in the process. I remain friends with every single one of them today.

But that is not always the case. Sometimes friends, family members, and/or acquaintances won't understand. It is not our responsibility to make them understand or sacrifice our wellbeing to simply show up. It *is* our responsibility to give a respectful response in as little or as much as one feels comfortable with. Not being physically present at an event dedicated to celebrating a child is in no way, shape, or form a denial of the incredible gift of new life that child is. It is not selfish. It is simply an acknowledgement of the importance of mental and emotional health; an act of self-care– just as counseling is. Finding a good, qualified counselor has been life-changing for me in multiple areas of my life.

Politely declining invitations has become more natural for me over the years. What has become harder is the extent of differences realized between our family and others that keep growing. The call to grow a family is beautiful—otherwise the inability to do so wouldn't hurt so much. Naturally, by extension of that, the more children others have, the farther apart our daily routines, conversation topics, and weekend plans become. Without intentional actions by both parties, relationships grow apart.

Both joys and the more rare, obvious tragedies related to new babies tend to, rightfully so, bring women together with great compassion and unwavering support. But the tragedy of new life never formed–and often life that never leaves the womb–slips through the cracks because it is suffered in silence; often unseen behind closed doors. Often forgotten.

We tend to mask the pain well and even become okay with our unexpected life circumstance, but the longing for community doesn't go away. No matter the source of anyone's pain, the longing to be seen doesn't change.

Some people would rather not talk about it, but I think it's more realistic to assume that they've gotten used to not being understood. It doesn't always feel emotionally safe. But you don't have to understand what the tragedy feels like to connect with the one who has been hurt by it.

The truth of the matter that no one likes to admit is that none of us understand what anybody else is going through until we walk in their shoes. Even if we find somebody trying to steer the same type of ship, we will never completely understand every unique person's experience. This is where *charity* and empathy come into play. If you remember from a few of our earlier conversations, charity, or love, is an act of the will that is often very difficult, but also very rewarding. And I am not sure whom I found it more difficult to choose love for: God on my most difficult day, or fertile women on every single day of my infertile life! But we can really only expect so much from other people who, through no fault of their own, don't have the same soul crushing concerns on their mind.

My dear friend, Emily @*totalwhine*, shared something on Instagram that I really connected with and find applicable here, even though she was talking about something completely unrelated like getting frustrated when distracted by children during prayer:

"I recently read a story about St. Mother Teresa told by a priest who knew and worked with her for years. He tells what he saw unfold when a photographer interrupted her during a rosary. It has changed the way I think about my prayer life amidst having toddlers...

'[S]he looked up [from prayer] and welcomed him with a radiant smile. Her attention now belonged entirely to [him]. He presented his business and left the chapel. Before he was even outside, Mother Teresa was already completely and utterly immersed again in prayer.

What moved me so much about this short scene was that Mother Teresa gave not even the slightest indication of displeasure or annoyance. On the contrary, it was as though the photographer had brought her a present by disturbing her at prayer. Only later did I understand that Jesus Himself was so present for [her] in the people she met that she–coming out of prayer, and thus out of a lively conversation with Jesus–simply shifted from Jesus to Jesus."
-<u>Mother Teresa of Calcutta: A Personal Portrait</u> by Leo Maasburg[8]

Ever since I read that post and regardless of the source of my frustration, I have been repeating those wisdom-filled words to myself: "from Jesus to Jesus," "From Jesus to Jesus," attempting to truly search for and connect with Jesus in every person. The same God that I chose to love on my worst day ever is the same Jesus that is in every person that hurts, frustrates, or angers me. Finding Jesus in every person really does change things.

No one enjoys feeling the crushing pressure of reminders of what you so desperately desire but do not have. But my spiritual director recently pointed out to me that he might actually be worried if I *wasn't* having such reactions of sadness and longing in response to the goodness of pregnancy. That reaction is a quite normal reflection of the absence, or loss of, something deeply meaningful and very, very good.

"Us"
I am grateful that God has put people in my life to help me transition my *"them"* attitude into an *"us"* attitude. Sometimes it is *actually* really easy to see Jesus in others. There are a few people in my life, both fertile and infertile, who have truly recognized my struggle and found a way to comfort me, addressing my needs in ways I couldn't have initially expressed a need for.

I knew I needed distance, but beyond that, I couldn't necessarily identify and verbalize *how* loved ones could help if they wanted to. Many people wonder what they can do to help in these situations. I have elaborated on a list below using examples of what others have done to uplift me. These have been game changers for my mental and emotional health. Consider these suggestions for couples who suffer with secondary infertility as well!

> **1. Be sensitive with announcements.** A couple of friends texted me to ask how they could respectfully deliver the news of a new pregnancy that would be easiest for me to receive. I considered this to be very thoughtful! For me, I found that receiving the news via

a text message allowed me to deal with my emotions privately, but still express sincere congratulations.

Sidenotes: If you're making a public announcement on Facebook, etc. and want to make it extra special, go to town. A little personal head's up ahead of time can ease the blow. When sending a private text message, *please* don't try and make it extra super cute and cryptic with any kind of picture, video, riddle, or something. It puts pressure on us to give some sort of excited reaction to news that is often hard to hear. Being straightforward will be much more helpful. Please know this doesn't mean we aren't very happy for you.

If you are making a big surprise announcement of pregnancy or gender reveal at an in-person party, it would likely mean a lot if you considered anyone present who might be sensitive to the news (even if they have been dealing with the struggle for years!) and give them a head's up beforehand. Being caught in the middle of that kind of excitement with nowhere to hide raw emotions could be devastating and stick with us for days or weeks.

2. So. Many. Announcements! Y'all. Recently, a few of my friends reached out with a gesture I never could've imagined would have been so healing for me. There have been a lot of pregnancy announcements in my friendship circle lately and one was particularly hard because of the way it was delivered. Three girlfriends of mine independently texted me with a, "Hey, I know there have been a lot of announcements lately. You have been on my heart. Are you okay?" Or "How are you doing? I just want you to know I've been thinking about you." Wow, was I touched! This acknowledgement of my pain made me feel seen when I had been struggling with such a sense of isolation.

3. Tell us that you're praying for us. Friends and acquaintances have consistently assured us of their prayers, even as years have passed. It's simple, but serves as a kind gesture to let us know we haven't been forgotten.

4. Limit pregnancy and baby talk. Discussions about pregnancies, birthing, babies, and schooling are all very good, but it is best to be done when surrounded by people who are familiar with the same situations. If there is an infertile woman present, chances are that she is struggling and hiding it well. It may be business as usual for you, but this could affect her for the next several weeks. It may not always be obvious, but please try to be aware of your surroundings and know your audience.

5. If adoption is sought, get excited. We have received an overwhelming amount of heartwarming encouragement and support throughout the process of adoption from close friends and acquaintances. I don't think I have encountered one person who has not made me feel as though they, too, consider Bella to be an equally important member of our family. When we brought Bella home for the first time, we were greeted by a balloon on our mailbox and a decorated garage door. Another friend, Ashley, had even cleaned our living room and kitchen and left a little helpful gift & huge "welcome baby" balloon on the counter. This made us feel so special!

6. Celebrate the heck out of the child/children they do have. If a couple has multiple children and multiple friends with multiple children, they may become a bit tired with the whole tradition of celebrating kids' birthday parties. This is understandable. But for those who struggle with infertility and may have only one or two children, these celebrations tend to be cherished. Bella's birthday parties are very special to us and it means a lot when that is reflected in our friendships. This doesn't mean you always *have* to show up, but it is meaningful if you are able to at least respond to the invitation.

7. Hire a babysitter. Make an effort for date nights without kids with friends.

8. Get creative. My sister, Angela, organized an incredibly thoughtful and adorably themed surprise *surgery shower* prior to my fifth surgery. It was pure genius. All of my friends were receiving multiple baby showers while I was receiving multiple weeks of recovery, but without the baby. So, she gathered my closest friends together to shower me with love and goodies to lift my spirits. There were latex gloves filled with popcorn, pill bottles filled with jelly beans, a game of operation, and more. I received gifts of colorful ice packs, fun socks, decorative cups to keep me hydrated, snacks, and more. I am still touched by all the effort and creativity that was offered through that party. This idea may not connect with or be practical for everyone, so please think it through. But there is no limit to God's creativity if you want to do *something* special.

9. Handheld encouragement. Angela is ridiculous-ly creative and thoughtful. She and friends have also contributed favorite Saint quotes, Scripture readings, and touching sentiments which my sister organized into a beautiful cloth book to accompany me to my out of state surgeries for frequent reference.

10. Spiritual Bouquet. I also learned that I had been the recipient of a *spiritual bouquet*. This is an endearing gesture delivered by listing out various specific prayers and/or sacrifices that people have promised to offer for me and Chris.

**Do not forget the husbands. It is important to *not* forget the husband of someone who is having surgery and/or experiencing infertility. Since the woman is the one that carries the baby and may be dealing with cycle issues, and it is often harder for men to verbalize their feelings, they frequently get left behind. Also, don't forget that men can be infertile, too! Maybe *he* is the one that is struggling with an inability to procreate. It has meant a lot, at least in our situation, when the guys check in on Chris from time to time whether we are recovering from surgery or not.

11. Meal train! Another incredibly helpful action taken by friends and family has been providing meals for us during recoveries. It is not unusual for meal trains to be started for families after the birth of a child. Families who require a postoperative healing period are equally in need of this kind of help. Same goes for after adoption!

12. Be vulnerable. One friend shared vulnerably with me that she was really wrestling with our two opposite realities––she was fervently practicing NFP/fertility awareness to avoid pregnancy in an attempt to space her children and desperately wished she could share some of her fertility with me. She could not understand God's plan and hated to see me suffer. I was so touched by her willingness to step into my suffering and feel it with me, even just for a moment. That is an act of love that truly opened my heart to her opposite, but equally valid, struggle.

13. Share in their pain. If there is one thing we can do for the people we love who are suffering, it is this: Sit and suffer with them, even just for a moment. 1 Corinthians 25-27 says *"...so that there should be no division in the body, but that its parts should have equal concern for each other. If one part suffers, every part suffers with it; if one part is honored, every part rejoices with it."* Although it is almost always out of good intentions, don't try to fix or give advice. Sit and lend your heart for both the sad *and* the good!

14. Get excited about their passions! This last suggestion is another act of love that has truly uplifted me and drawn me even closer to friends or back into relationships that I had previously felt left out of due to my inability to relate to many topics discussed. It may be the most important thing on this list. Many women in my circle have many babies and although my first and most important baby, Bella, is most obvious, I also have many other babies which I have created and nursed to life. So, when anyone identifies, applauds, encourages, supports, or takes any amount of interest in any of the hard work I have put into my outreach, writing, rapping, teaching, speaking, or podcasting, it allows me to feel connected to and cared for by them. It truly gives me new life!

That goes both ways. It is just as important for me to support and encourage their gifts, talents, endeavors, and whatever. We need to make the interests of those close to us our interests, too. And I don't mean a fake pat on the back—we don't have to be throwing parades for the same causes to take a genuine interest in the gifts of the ones we love. Consider friends who aren't necessarily infertile, but are unmarried, or are simply unable to attempt achieving pregnancy despite a great desire to. Two close friends of mine who have serious medical reasons to avoid pregnancy are both being used by God to bring new life into the world in extraordinary and meaningful ways which, in turn, fills their hearts. Their ministries are their babies. Nothing makes a person light up more than talking about something, or someone, they are passionate about. When we do this, we are all fostering an abundance of Christ into this world.

As with my anger at God, I have come a long way with releasing the bitterness I have harbored towards other women. It takes repetitive efforts, but when I see what God has done with my life; with my infertility, I cannot *not* be grateful. I cannot wish I had it any other way. That gratitude has to extend to every new life that God creates. How can I be grateful for the new life that comes from within me and not from within someone else? Every single time God breathes new life into a little soul, it is an absolute miracle, not unlike the many miracles he has ordained in my own. This is something to remember when trudging through the rugged terrains of suffering, which can either leave us in despair or connect us with the cross of Christ. The choice is ours.

CHAPTER 12

Suffering

*"Next to my vocation, the greatest gift I have
is the pain I carry every day, because it forces
me to cling to Jesus."*
— *Mother Angelica*

THREE TRIPS TO THE EMERGENCY room for morphine, two to urgent care for Toradol injections, eleven surgeries, monthly narcotics, nausea, vomiting, countless hours writhing in bedsheets, the tub, and/or the bathroom floor, dramatic diet changes, planning life around a period, and sometimes daily anti-inflammatories—for many women, the emotional pain of infertility is only one side of the coin.

Undoubtedly, the underlying causes of my physical pain have purchased my ticket for infertility. It has been an interesting tango between the two sources (infertility and endometriosis) of my deepest suffering, both emotional *and* physical. The chronic physical pain that I have become all too familiar with is puzzling to me. It began when I was about twelve years old and worsened as I aged, sowing itself into my identity to a certain extent. I have experienced it for so long that it is what I know to be a part of life; even strangely comforting at times.

The pain has molded itself into a sort of cyclic monster I have learned to fear because even the strongest medicines available for personal use cannot control it. It isn't discomfort that just comes every once in a while. It is a freight train running at full speed and plowing into my body twelve times a year whether I'm ready for it or not. When you are at the mercy of such a ruthless beast of a disease, there is only one place to turn: Calvary.

No human has ever suffered as much as Christ during his crucifixion. Although He was fully man *and* fully God, He did not make Himself immune to any kind of suffering. He willingly stepped into many of our human experiences, making himself susceptible to the really good and the really hard. He, more than anyone, has not only the ability, but the intense desire to meet us right where we are, especially when where we are doesn't look so pretty.

Heb 2: 17-18 (NABRE) says *"[17] therefore, he had to become like his brothers in every way, that he might be a merciful and faithful high priest before God to expiate the sins of the people. [18] Because he himself was tested through what he suffered, he is able to help those who are being tested."*

Agonizing pain has a way of holding your thoughts captive. No one teaches you how to respond appropriately in those rare, extreme situations because, well, they are rare and many people don't know what to do. The best person to take our cues from is Jesus Himself. There are times when I'm simply trying to make it through to the next minute and find that the only thing I can focus on is the TV screen or my grip on the bed sheet. But there are also moments of pure inspiration when I am able to meet Christ at the foot of the cross. It takes concentration and effort, but sometimes I feel like I can reach out to

Him and press my cheek up against his bloody feet for some relief and comfort, sharing ever so slightly in His suffering. In light of this aspect, I am often able to view suffering as a privilege.

Mother Teresa said[9]: *"Suffering has to come because if you look at the cross, he has got his head bending down—he wants to kiss you—and he has both hands open wide—he wants to embrace you. He has his heart opened wide to receive you. Then when you feel miserable inside, look at the cross and you will know what is happening. Suffering, pain, sorrow, humiliation, feelings of loneliness, are nothing but the kiss of Jesus, a sign that you have come so close that he can kiss you...Suffering, pain, humiliation—this is the kiss of Jesus. At times you come so close to Jesus on the cross that he can kiss you..."*

That imagery is beautiful and everything, but when you are in the heat of suffering through [insert source here] and can barely hold it together, a more likely response would be a crass "Could you please tell Jesus to stop kissing me?!" And this is exactly how one woman reacted to Mother Teresa herself. So, she added: *"That suffering has to come that came in the life of Our Lady, that came in the life of Jesus—it has to come in our life also. Only never put on a long face. Suffering is a gift from God. It is between you and Jesus alone inside."*

There were many times that I felt *done* with all of it. But there is a depth that we can reach at some point where we no longer have the strength to hold onto our own will, and we are finally able to relax into the arms of Jesus Himself.

"On the Christian Meaning of Human Suffering"
To be *redeemed* means "to buy or pay off; clear by payment" (dictionary.com.) Human *redemption* was paid

for by one perfect Man, Christ, and through one specific experience of suffering and death. That suffering has *immeasurable* value. As we are called to imitate Christ, in His generosity, He has allowed us to take part in that Redemption. Pope St. John Paul II describes the perplexing benefit of joining our sufferings with Jesus on the Cross in his Apostolic letter, "Salvifici Doloris... on the Christian meaning of human suffering:[10]"

"In bringing about the Redemption through suffering, Christ has also raised human suffering to the level of the Redemption. Thus each man, in his suffering, can also become a sharer in the redemptive suffering of Christ."

"Therefore the Apostle [Paul] will also write in the Second Letter to the Corinthians: 'For as we share abundantly in Christ's sufferings, so through Christ we share abundantly in comfort too.'"
"Those who share in the sufferings of Christ are also called, through their own sufferings, to share in glory."

"Suffering as it were contains a special call to the virtue which man must exercise on his own part. And this is the virtue of perseverance in bearing whatever disturbs and causes harm. In doing this, the individual unleashes hope, which maintains in him the conviction that suffering will not get the better of him, that it will not deprive him of his dignity as a human being, a dignity linked to awareness of the meaning of life.

"In this Body [of Christ], Christ wishes to be united with every individual, and in a special way he is united with those who suffer."

What a unique experience of intimacy it is to unite our suffering with Christ, as it was through *His* greatest suffering that He redeemed the world! When our discomforts are useless, they are a source of complaint. But when our suffering has a purpose, it is of great use to ourselves, our family, Christ, the Church, and the world.

"...suffering also has a special value in the eyes of the Church. It is something good, before which the Church bows down in reverence with all the depth of her faith in the Redemption. She likewise bows down with all the depth of that faith with which she embraces within herself the inexpressible mystery of the Body of Christ."

"This is the meaning of suffering, which is truly supernatural and at the same time human. It is supernatural because it is rooted in the divine mystery of the Redemption of the world, and it is likewise deeply human, because in it the person discovers himself, his own humanity, his own dignity, his own mission."

"The Church bows down in reverence" to our suffering. Doesn't that put a different spin on the agonies we encounter throughout life? Our perspectives matter! How we choose to respond to the hardships of life, big and small, will determine its effects on us. Suffering certainly has the capacity to break us down, but that doesn't have to be a bad thing. It shaves off the rough edges of sin and dysfunction to uncover the human underneath. It is often this painful process that allows us to fully discover ourselves, and thus fully donate ourselves to serve Christ within the world.

Useful
Before I knew my friend Emily, she encountered what she describes as an impossibly scary and isolating situation which became a dramatic test of her faith. At the time, she would've likened NFP to a natural form of birth control, putting all her stock in that avoiding pregnancy option, thanks to poor NFP/fertility awareness education. She

was a little shaken when an NFP pregnancy surprised her and her new husband not long after they got married. Things became more serious when she discovered she would need a C section since her baby was full breech. Childbirth wouldn't be "natural" for her like she had hoped, but would require major surgery. In an attempt to limit the amount of lifetime C-sections which carry their own severe risks, her doctor recommended that she avoid pregnancy for at least nine months. This, in combination with the NFP fail and the hormonal acrobatics of postpartum, delivered a variety of challenges.

She made a significant emotional and financial investment into a new fertility awareness method, hoping that the steep costs would allow her and her husband to delay another pregnancy as medically prescribed. So, when that little positive sign popped up on a pregnancy test a mere seven months later with a newborn already in tow, she was met with complete spiritual and emotional desolation. She was now faced with another C-section when she hadn't emotionally, psychologically, or physically processed the trauma of the first, another NFP fail, and another young child.

Her trust in God flew out the window while any sense of peace, comfort, or control snuck out the back door as she experienced her own dark night of the soul. But she chose to remain grounded in her faith despite feeling nothing from or for her Creator, something that she called "falling back on faithfulness." She explains that, after God turned the lights back on in her soul, she realized that she had experienced precisely what Mother Teresa described: the painful kiss of Jesus. The darkness was an invitation to a deeper intimacy with Christ crucified, which gave birth to a deeper understanding of suffering and an unquenchable desire to step into the pain of others who carry their own unique crosses. Her whole experience of darkness transformed her outlook on suffering, faith, and even fertility awareness. It made her better.

Suffering can cut just as deep and be equally as purposeful whether it is physical, psychological, or emotional. Christ experienced all of it first and worst. He is the ideal person to teach us *how to* suffer well and *how* to bring meaning into it. He desires peace and joy for all of us, even as we suffer great trials.

If you look to Scripture for the example of his suffering, death, and Resurrection, you will see a counter-cultural approach to carrying a cross: willingness. For me, it was *willingness* that made a big difference. We hear during the consecration at each Mass that *"[Christ] willingly entered into His passion..."* No one forced him to carry His cross. He took it up on His own accord.

Matthew 26:39 (NABRE) says, *"[39] He advanced a little and fell prostrate in prayer, saying, "My Father,[a] if it is possible, let this cup pass from me; yet, not as I will, but as you will."*

We hear Our Blessed Mother Mary echo the same sentiment in her infamous Fiat in Luke 1:38 (NABRE): *"[38] Mary said, "Behold, I am the handmaid of the Lord. May it be done to me according to your word..."*

It may not be very well understood by the vast majority of humanity, but the recommended response to suffering is spelled out pretty clearly in Scripture. The first and second holiest people that have ever existed on earth and now dwell in the ultimate glory of heaven teach us how to suffer well––in a way that doesn't remove pain, but allows us to experience growth from it. As I stopped viewing my suffering as something being done to me and started to explore it, I began to find it useful and transformative.

"Useful" is the key word, here, which my father has taught me a lot about. My dad is an interesting combination of wit and wisdom tucked behind a very serious-looking exterior. He tends to be very quiet, which can easily lend one to assume a snobby perception of him. If you are familiar with "RBF," you are familiar with my dad's face. We call it RGF: "Resting Grumpaw Face." Nevertheless, the man knows his Catholic Church teaching, scripture, and any other kind of Catholic reading material or podcast personality.

During a particularly challenging time in my life, he dropped an incredibly ancient-looking book onto the table in front of me and said, "I think you will find this useful." He had already neatly underlined the juiciest bits of wisdom in it, bookmarked on about twenty different pages, and I was *all in*.

In "The Practice of the Love of Jesus Christ[11]," St. Alphonsus Ligouri explains:

"Solomon says, 'One who is slow to anger is better than the mighty' (Prov 16:32). God is pleased by persons who practice mortification by fasting, hair shirts, and disciplines, because of the courage displayed in such mortifications; but he is much more pleased by those who have the courage to bear patiently and cheerfully the crosses that God sends them.

St. Francis de Sales said, 'The mortifications that come to us from God, or from fellow humans with God's permission, are always more precious than those born from our own will. It is a general rule that the less our choice is involved, the more pleased God is, and the greater profit for ourselves.'

St. Teresa of Avila taught the same thing: 'We gain more in one day from the afflictions visited on us by God or our neighbor than from ten years of self-inflicted suffering.'"

"Better than ten years of self-inflicted suffering!" Did I read that correctly? I figured that referring to my suffering as a "privilege" in the beginning of this chapter might provoke crazy eyes in my general direction from some readers, but there is truth buried behind those very words! St. Teresa of Avila said that, *"You pay God a compliment by asking great things of Him."* Well, I don't think it is far off to turn that around and suggest that God, too, pays us a compliment by asking great things of us.

Most of us can look at our lives and identify how some struggles have made us better and stronger, even enriching us. You can usually recognize those individuals who haven't experienced much challenge in their lives (yet––suffering will find all of us in one form or another) and are *not* necessarily better for it. Maybe those same people *have* been introduced to suffering but chose to run the other way in hopes of escaping it. Granted, I have fallen on my face many times despite trying to suffer well, but I am better and more "alive" because of those personal challenges.

There are three words tattooed in my brain (by the ultimate graffiti artist of the Holy Spirit) as analogous to the word suffering: "depth of life." This is how I view it. When one talks about "depth of color" or "clarity" in a photograph, for example, it refers to the number of bits or pixels present. The more bits or pixels that exist per area, the more vibrant and crystal clear the picture is. This is what suffering has done for me. It actually has the capacity to unlock new intensities and experiences of life when we give it the chance.

This idea inspired some of my lyrics in the last verse of "Battle Wounds:"

There's life in pain–don't stay in the darkness
Better rise from ash! Joy is mine to harness
From dead man walkin' to wise man talkin'
Life is mine to seize when I stay on my knees
I was a fool to think that he was mine to taunt–
Love him hard even if I don't get what I want
Ride or die, this has allowed you and me
To lock up hopelessness and throw away that key

I don't want to forget the pain that got me here
Wearing these wounds destroys my fear
If I ever forget, please get remindin'
My scars will sparkle like diamonds
I don't want to forget the pain that got me here
Wearing these wounds destroys my fear
Nobody can tell me that it wasn't worth the fight
Every scar on my skin is placed just right

Ten stripes deep–they've made me who I am
Eleven laps on this track–but I. Still. Stand.

It's true that I wouldn't need the joy and cathartic release of writing and rapping if I hadn't experienced the physical impairments and infertility in the first place. But without that pain I also wouldn't have experienced this depth of life unknown to me before. I would *not* have had the inspiration or drive to dig into these talents now breathing life into the desires of my heart. There is something about pain that makes us come alive! It has the capacity to motivate us to fight not just for ourselves, but for others as well.

Mission

Part of the inspiration for anything I do is driven by helping other women to cope with infertility and other sufferings, choose God, and/or get appropriate medical help efficiently. God often uses the sufferings of some to help others, sometimes bringing life-changing results.

The suffering my friend, Emily, lived through as a result of those two unplanned pregnancies and poor fertility awareness education opened her eyes to many of the real needs that multitudes of women and couples have. So, she was inspired to do something about it. She created a website and started a blog called "total whine," where she "w(h)ines" about the real-life challenges of parenting, marriage, sex, faith, NFP/fertility awareness, and more. In her own words, "I love my Catholic faith, and believe that the greatest way to evangelize is to live it joyfully AND honestly...humor and honesty are my tools. Solidarity is my goal. Welcome to my gloves-off musings on living the faith. Pour a dram and dive on in!" And let me tell you, she has struck a harmonious chord with countless women.

Her authentic approach to these uncommonly discussed topics have truly resonated with women everywhere who frequently end up in her inbox with a, "This is exactly how I feel. Thank you so much for talking about this" and more of, "You've taught me so much about [this thing] that I didn't think anyone else would understand." She uncovered a vast unfilled space where there was a longing for community and continues to make the appropriate connections between people, faith, knowledge, and real life as a rapidly growing Catholic social media influencer.

This "W(h)iner-in-Chief" has grown tremend-ously from her suffering, unlocking a mission that God designed perfectly for her. This is only one of the many profound ways that she brings new life into the world in addition to her two tiny and beautiful little humans.

She has, essentially:
- Experienced deep pain and anger at God
- Overcome a huge test of faith
- Learned of some real-life gaps that needed filling through the process
- Used her experience to fill those gaps
- Has in-turn been incredibly fulfilled by discovering one of her God-given life missions.

This has provided her with a sense of peace and satisfaction that is ongoing as she continuously uses the gifts God has given her to serve others. What I have experienced as a result of my own unique sufferings has been similar. Remember one of the quotes from Pope St. JP II's Salvifici Doloris[10]: *"Those who share in the sufferings of Christ are also called, through their own sufferings, to share in glory."* He can not only transform the ugliest of life experiences into something beautiful, but touch the hearts of many others through it.

Think about how many lives are touched by adoption, which is often the result of an unplanned pregnancy: the adoptive parents, the child, the birth mother, the associated families and friends, and even future generations. Think about how many foundations and movements to promote education were started due to an unfortunate experience of suffering by a loved one. I'm not suggesting that we must create successful public campaigns to make our suffering useful! We are simply called to be open to whatever God is asking of us by becoming moldable and docile to His plans. Maybe we are being called to offer our suffering up for someone else in need or maybe the experience itself will help us to grow in love and empathy. Maybe there is simply something important God wants us to learn. Whether we have the foresight to see the potential good our struggles can bring or not, they are bountiful. With our trust and permission, God will multiply His goodness from life's painful experiences.

We learn who we really are when we are broken down by life's challenges. This provides us with ample opportunities to choose love no matter how unexpected and inconvenient these challenges become. And God knows we all get plenty of chances to practice. The next road bump Chris and I encountered gave us quite the wedding weekend surprise!

CHAPTER 13

Sex & Marriage

"Intense love does not measure, it just gives."
— Saint Theresa of Calcutta

CHRIS AND I PROMISED FOREVER to each other on another warm New Orleans day that should've been cold. Our wedding also took place on the only January day that it didn't rain in our hometown in 2013, which I thought was pretty cool. I always feared that I'd be riddled with anxiety on that special day in anticipation of so many big changes happening all at once. My I do's meant fully committing myself until death, merging finances, moving in with a boy, sharing a fridge, a bathroom, and a bed, *and* having sex for the first time. And then many more times after that.

Thankfully, God graced me with an unexplainable peace that was apparently palpable as my friends began to comment on how notably calm I appeared that entire day. It felt like a confirmation for the man I was choosing to love in good times, and especially in the bad. I don't care if you're infertile, fertile, poor, rich, or running from an escaped convict. No marriage is perfect. All should fluctuate between periods of romance and disillusionment, and hopefully increasing periods of true joy. The quality of our relationships is not measured by each period of romance, but in our ability to choose one another when it is flat out hard. Chris taught me how to do that.

We were fortunate enough to stay at the Ritz-Carlton in downtown New Orleans for an incredible first two nights as Mr. and Mrs. Bruno, thanks to a family friend. As one of their many attentions to detail, they gifted us with a tall, narrow, luxurious glass of bubble bath wearing a fancy white key pendant necklace to celebrate our special occasion. We used that bottle of bubbles to explore each other in new ways which, unfortunately, gave way to new problems we were previously unaware of.

Intercourse may be slightly uncomfortable the first time, but I've recently learned from an experienced pelvic floor physical therapist that it should never be painful. This shocked me as I considered the many different ways in which sex *has* hurt over the years, and how I've always assumed that it was something I should just deal with––yet another women's health issue that needs major attention! It was that inaugural attempt that was the worst, as all that anticipation was built up only to take a sharp nose dive. With practice, the act of that sacred union did become more bearable over the next couple of weeks, but remained uncomfortable––even momentarily excruciating at times.

It turns out that painful intercourse can be a side effect of endometriosis, that inflammatory condition that produces scar tissue and adhesions within the pelvic cavity that I told you about several chapters ago. It had been previously spotted on my uterus, ovaries, and bowel, organs that are all located very close to each other within a space that becomes even more intimate during sex. I would later learn that the frequent pain I had throughout the years caused me to tense up regularly, which taught my entire pelvic floor to remain tight and angry. Endometriosis just keeps on giving...

It wasn't until after our ninth wedding anniversary that I was finally diagnosed with a condition called vaginismus, defined as a "painful spasmodic contraction of the vagina in response to physical contact or pressure (especially in sexual intercourse)," according to the dictionary on my iphone. Since I had never experienced sex in the first place, I didn't know what it was supposed to feel like. But I certainly didn't expect what is intended to unite spouses in passionate excitement to physically hurt *so* much. I expected it to do the opposite.

So, I saved sex for marriage and––surprise!––it's not enjoyable, like, at all. They don't typically prepare you for that in marriage prep. Neither of us were sure how to mentally, spiritually, or physically approach this situation. Chris hated to cause so much pain and I tried to manage it as much as possible (something I should not have done, in case you were wondering) because I desired to be intimate with him *and* for him to enjoy it–a strange dynamic for this newly-married couple.

Theology of...Painful Sex?
To be clear, help should be sought if you are experiencing any kind of consistent pain with intercourse. God has designed sex to be an incredible act of unity and fruitfulness of which pleasure is a beautiful and integral part. We are meant to have *positive pelvic experiences*, as my friend Emily puts it. It is good to seek help to restore this function of intercourse. Consult a pelvic floor physical therapist, physician, and/or a counselor for help. Talk to your husband about it. In the meantime, let's take a deep dive into this underdiscussed topic of painful sex.

About seven months after we tied the knot, we were fortunate enough to attend a one-day marriage retreat in Houma, Louisiana, offered by Christopher West. I was pumped! Obviously, the Theology of the Body is a topic through which he is able to beautifully articulate God's plan for sex and marriage. His talks were brilliant, as usual, but mentioned nothing specifically related to my concerns. I was dying to know what he might have to say about when sex is painful.

I asked one of his associates how I might be able to ask him this important question. He was very kind, offering to pass an email over to Mr. West for me and I was pleasantly surprised when he wrote back. I was touched that he responded at all, but I was moved (ok, this was definitely a fan-girl moment) by the in-depth, personal, and compassionate words he had to offer:

"You asked what God asks you to do in this situation and if you were looking at it the right way. I do believe this is an opportunity for both of you to grow in love of one another and to find deep intimacy with Christ in your sufferings. This is, indeed, a 'great mystery' that Christ consummates his marriage on what St. Augustine called 'the marriage bed of the cross'...

A bed of suffering. It seems to me that you have a very intimate share in that suffering. It is certainly a fruitful suffering united to Jesus.

I can't help but notice your name as the name of the 'woman' who stood at the foot of Christ's cross receiving that 'sword through her heart' prophesied in Scripture. I would urge you to draw close to Mary in your sufferings. She will teach you the way of remaining 'open' to whatever cross Christ may ask you to carry.

Mary, you are very, very close to Jesus and Mary in this suffering you bear...never forget that the 'agony' Christ allows in our lives is all 'training' for the ecstasy he has in store for us."
*He also recommended seeking medical help

"Christ consummates his marriage on...the marriage bed of the cross." Obviously, Jesus did not consummate a marriage in the sense you and I are used to. A Christian marriage between a man and a woman on earth is in imitation of Christ being "wed" to His bride, the Church and not a woman. The expression of *the marriage bed of the cross* is used to describe that profound moment of union between Christ and the Church as He sacrificed His life for her on the cross––an incredibly meaningful *and fruitful* moment of agony.

Painful intercourse and the abstinence that results in the process of healing is not what God planned or what we expect. It is, indeed, another source of suffering, and another opportunity to be drawn close into the heart of Christ. As you are well aware, that act of love offered by Christ on the cross gave birth to our salvation and paved the way for the Holy Spirit to set the world on fire as the Apostles spread the good news throughout the world. In like form, our expression of love through the act of intercourse, and our resolve to love each other through difficult seasons of healing and painful periods of abstinence, has great capacity to bear fruit.

I doubt Mr. West had any idea how profoundly this message would resonate within my heart and then translate to far more than the physical discomfort of sex! He was unaware of the intense cramps I experienced regularly, the surgeries I already had, and the surgeries that were yet to come, yet the message applies to all of it.

His thoughts echo everything that Christ teaches us about suffering, how He draws us in during those difficult times, and how He so generously shares His own mother to lift our chin so we can fix our gaze upon Himself. It was a necessary and gentle reminder of how fiercely Christ's eyes had already been fixed on me. No matter the source, God is pleased to share intimately in all of our sufferings. The pleasure of sex is good and is intended by its Designer, but it can't be compared to the euphoria of heaven that our earthly troubles prepare us for. I certainly didn't apply this message perfectly, but it did give me hope.

But this brings up another interesting conversation about the level at which sex has been elevated to in our culture and can have a great impact on how we live out this Sacrament. Sex is practically coveted by many who don't understand what it means to love authentically. It has become an activity that some believe is silly to save for the lifetime commitment of marriage, and that others are forced to have whether overtly or implicitly through guilt—even within some marriages. Our society has championed unrestricted sex to the detriment of pre-born babies, respect for women of all ages, and actual women empowerment. Some dismiss the unitive purpose and elevate the procreative purpose, or the other way around. It is no surprise that so many of us feel empty, confused, and unloved.

Our culture generally promotes service of self, but it is selfishness that we ought to be trying to push out of the bedroom. Sex was designed to unite a man and a woman who have promised forever to each other and who remain open to welcoming the new life that unity fosters in any and all of its forms. It is precisely this act of making a complete and total self-gift to the other, uniting body, mind, and spirit, the whole person, that provides our most complete fulfillment.

Sexual intimacy is not limited to contact with the genitals. It's contact with the *whole* human person. It is spiritual, creative, physical (both within and without the context of sex), emotional, artistic, communicative, recreational, and every other way that one can fathom growing in intimacy with the one we have chosen to love. Pleasure alone does not make "good sex." It is the willingness of the couple to continue to work on uniting their whole selves to one another that results in pleasure in all aspects of their relationship. Lloyd and Jan Tate add that "It is the depth of communication that sets the pulse of the marriage." It is not the degree to which we experience sexual satisfaction.

If sex had been a major focus and identity of our relationship, what might it have done to us when intercourse didn't turn out as expected? What would our relationship be like through long periods of abstinence? If we had taken our culture's advice on sex, would we have experienced the satisfaction of authentic love in good times and in bad? Would I be capable of finding such incredible joy through my suffering?

Same Bubbles. Different Scenario.
That fancy bottle of bubbles that we received from the Ritz not long after we exchanged vows has been rarely used since that weekend which brought new forms of joy and pain. It became a beautiful and nostalgic decoration around our bathtub at home.

When I picture our tub, I picture that bottle, which now encapsulates an even greater significance because of a newer experience we had. My pain had gotten bad again and the medication wasn't kicking in, so it was time to get into the tub. Chris told me to stay on the couch until he could prepare the bath water for me. When the time came, he carefully helped me into the bathroom and into the tub, where the hot water provided some relief instantly.

Finally able to relax a little, I laid there and remained as still as possible in an effort to avoid disturbing my cyclic monster. Chris immediately grabbed that precious bottle of bubbles from our wedding night and poured it all around me, its aroma instantly tickling my nose.

Same bubbles. Very different scenario.

That precious bottle decorated our bathtub for years without being touched. In my head, it had become a prized reminder of our first few nights as husband and wife and should only be used for the most special of occasions. This ended up becoming one of them. After settling the bottle back into its treasured spot, he found some bath salts I didn't even know we had and sprinkled them into the water as well. He sat next to me and held my hand from the other side of the tub.

The hot water felt good but eventually made me feel so hot that I felt like I needed to get out. Chris insisted that I stay and began to fan me with two thick Creighton charts that were lying near the sink. A smile broke through the stoic expression on my face as I uttered, "This is marriage..." and he smiled, too. My body and fertility betrayed me with pain and dysfunction, but my heart was full and my spirit was content, even joyful. A similar scenario was repeated less than two weeks later.

On a night in which I was in great physical pain, both of us bearing hearts with dreams of fertility crushed, one of us fully clothed and clutching my hand, and no orgasm in sight, we had a fulfilling sexual experience. By the grace of God, we were able to crumple up the distorted meaning of sexual intimacy fed to us by our culture, applying it to instant gratification alone, and flush it down the drain.

My whole person connected with his whole person. I was open and completely vulnerable as Chris made a complete and sincere gift of himself to me. I received that gift and reciprocated it back to him in my gratitude and sincere appreciation in as much as I was able to in that moment. We both experienced the pleasure of a deeper intimacy.
Clearly, this is no substitute for sexual intercourse, but it broadens a limited concept of sexual fulfillment. Mind-blowing, toe-curling sex is the goal. It *is* how God designed a married couple to experience intercourse, but it is unlikely that that will be every person's experience every single time. Sex won't always be perfect and for various reasons. Sometimes sex won't happen at all. It doesn't mean a couple can't still have satisfying sexual experiences. It does not mean their marriage is crippled. It means there is room for physical, spiritual, and/or emotional healing. It means that we are human and that sex–and self control–is an opportunity to grow in love and union with our spouse *and Christ* no matter the circumstances.

Physically pleasurable sex is very good, and should be sought for married couples! But it is possible to be happy, content, intimate, and satisfied when sex is not perfect, or even present at all.

This is Marriage
Not long after this memorable and, strangely, treasured experience, we celebrated a special day. I was still in a lot of pain, so we approached our wedding anniversary

differently than we are usually able to, but I had never felt more intimately loved by or connected to my husband, who continues to choose me at my lowest.

This has transformed my understanding of sexuality.

For many infertile couples, there is a point at which sex becomes a chore. God designed each act of intercourse with two primary purposes—unitive and openness to new life in any of its forms. As months, and then years, pass without that treasured conception, it's almost as if that unitive purpose unintentionally fades off slowly into the background. A baby becomes minimized to a goal rather than the result of the self-donation of love between husband and wife. Sex becomes a means to an end. When sex ceases being a choice two people make to renew their vows, it also ceases growth in intimacy. There is nothing wrong with fertility-focused intercourse, but when the sole purpose of intercourse becomes conception, we lose sight of our spouse.

The challenge is to maintain those twofold purposes of sex no matter the circumstances. Whether there is a hyper focus on having a baby *or* any measure of excluding new life, the unitive aspect of the embrace is undermined. Our goal should be to maintain sex as a celebration of love. It is not an end in and of itself, but a celebration of the whole relationship. That is what makes us capable of bearing fruit – not merely the biological ability to produce a child.

Having our priorities in the right order is paramount. My mom loves to say, *"I am third; God first, others second, and myself third."* That number two spot is reserved for our spouse. A quick and easy way to check ourselves is to take an honest look at where having a baby ranks on the list––whether we're infertile or not. This is a sure-fire way to help discern IVF, too.

Infertility can drain us in multiple different areas of life––physical, emotional, relational, marital. Grasping the concept of sex for how it was intended to be celebrated and loving our spouse authentically will ease some of that added stress.

The Pulse for Marriage
I have found the goodness of life not so much to be in the great culmination of all the things I want or expect, but in how I overcome and triumph over each struggle and tragedy. God has made the most beautiful creations come from each one. It has been an honor to be able to share this and all we have learned very early on in marriage with our engaged couples as marriage prep mentors. My favorite piece of experience to share with them is the value that difficulties in life and marriage can bring.

When imagining what married life will be like, many of us envision some variation of a white picket fence, glorious snuggles, and maybe even frolicking in fields of daisies. They don't adorn greeting cards of congratulations with the growing pains of suffering, but it is precisely the combination of our joys and our growth through struggles that has made my marriage so sweet. Difficulties can, and should, become doorways to intimacy.

As explained in regards to spiritual parenthood, this was a ministry we did not plan for. It wasn't even on our radar because what married couple thinks they are qualified to mentor engaged couples after only five years? But because we were asked by some good friends, we took some time to think about it and ask God if this was what He wanted. Four couples later, it has made a palpable difference in the strength and intimacy of our relationship, and has become a beautiful source of new life. What qualifies a couple to be a mentor couple is their openness to God, His plan for their lives, their decision to be faithful to the Sacrament, and willingness to be vulnerable with the couples He entrusts them with.

The beauty about being in the mentor position is that we are frequently studying the material in an effort to present the information well to our engaged couples. This has allowed us to truly internalize many beautiful Church teachings and lessons about the Sacrament and relationships. We have learned the irreplaceable value of good, deep communication, and growth in intimacy in all of its forms. Our goal is to make more of an effort to share our whole selves—fears, joys, interests, thoughts, etc. to encounter more of the other person. We can never stop learning about each other. In the movie "Fireproof," Kirk Cameron's character learns this valuable lesson through the idea of "studying" his spouse: *"When the man is trying to win the heart of a woman, he studies her. He learns her likes and dislikes, habits and hobbies... If the amount he studied her before he married her was equal to a high school degree, he should continue to learn about her until he gains a college degree, a Master's degree, and ultimately, a Doctorate degree. It is a lifelong journey that draws his heart ever closer to hers."*

When our emotional, communicative, and spiritual muscles are working well, it enhances the depth of our sexual experience, which if you remember, is an experience of the whole person and not just the "special" parts.

Lloyd and Jan Tate (creators of our marriage prep program and resident marriage all stars) explain that:

"The depth and openness of communication set the pulse of the marriage relationship", and that "the sexual relationship is not a separate and distinct aspect of your marriage; it is an extension of your whole relationship and an expression of your unity and intimacy...intended to be a celebration of the emotional and spiritual intimacy the couple is experiencing in all aspects of their relationship."

In other words: the better the emotional and spiritual intimacy, the better the sex. Like Lloyd Tate says, "I would venture to say that that is not how sex was described to you as an adolescent!" The way God has designed sex is mind-blowingly awesome to an extent that is sometimes hard to comprehend. Neither marriage nor sex tends to turn out exactly how we expect and for a number of reasons. But that's why authentic love is so important! It doesn't matter what hiccup or roadblock is headed our way because love is a choice we can make always and forever and no matter what. Chris and I's next unexpected "adventure" would deliver even bigger challenges. If you were around when I began to encounter what came next, you might have even referred to me as a "hot mess"--both figuratively and literally.

CHAPTER 14

Hot Mess

"If a man wishes to be sure of the road he treads on, he must close his eyes and walk in the dark."
— *Saint John of the Cross*

LATE LAST YEAR, I WAS in the middle of presenting a Creighton Model Introductory Session in my home office to a newly engaged couple when I suddenly felt a steep rise in temperature. My skin was damp and clammy at first, then it began to release larger drops of moisture, typically referred to as *sweat*. I went from sitting comfortably inside of my air-conditioned home to sweating and questioning the functionality of the AC in a matter of seconds. It was so unexpectedly jarring that I lost my place in the presentation and asked the couple "Did it just get really hot in here?" thinking something might be wrong with the AC.

With a confused look on their faces, they exchanged a quick and awkward glance in response to the crazy lady sitting in front of them and responded, "Hmm, no?" Then I had to conceal my emotions as I suddenly connected the dots. This was not the first time I experienced hot flashes, but it was the first time I experienced them without being on Clomid, a medication commonly used to induce ovulation. I picked my heart back up off the floor and stumbled through the rest of the presentation.

About three or four years prior to that night was the first time I felt like I was being set on fire internally, but it didn't bother me because I knew it was a response to the medication I was taking. I didn't want to think about what this could possibly mean, so I tried to ignore it. But the hot flashes continued. The very next cycle was extra long, followed by two very short cycles, and this was all extremely unusual––even for me. For as much trouble as my period gave me, my cycles were pretty consistent. At the time, I was seeing my local NaPro medical consultant and friend, Dr. Susan Caldwell, for follow ups every other month. When she took a look at my chart and saw this weird sequence, she uttered a few words that nearly knocked me off my feet: "This looks like perimenopause."

Uhhhhhhhhhhhhhhhh, excuse me whaaa? Menopause? Hello? I was thirty-one years old! IS THIS THING ON!? I was only fifteen like…sixteen years ago. I got married only six birthdays ago. And did I mention that I HAVEN'T BEEN PREGNANT YET? Shouldn't I have at least fifteen years to try? I'm not ready, or old enough, to be in menopause! If you've seen that infamous 2013 Jim Mora (Colts head coach at the time) post-game press conference, then you know exactly how I uttered the word "menopause?!"–– "Playoffs?! What you talkin' about? You kidding me? I just hope we can win a game!"

For years I had been cautiously preparing for someone to tell me that I was in need of a hysterectomy, but *that* was going to be a *choice*. Early menopause was nowhere near my radar. This was different. It was a sucker-punch to the gut that I did not see coming.

This introduced a new kind of healing that would need to take place. It was all so incredibly confusing that I didn't even understand how to feel. One word that kept coming to mind to describe this new feeling was "humiliated" because I am so young and I only knew of menopause to be experienced by women much older than me.

Putting the fertility aspect aside, how would this change how I feel each day? How would this effect my libido? My weight? My sleep? I also felt "embarrassed," even when I was all alone and within the privacy of my own emotions. It was so hard to wrap my head around this. My husband, who was incredibly supportive and understanding, was the only one who knew that this was going on for a while. I eventually told a few close friends and family members who I knew would receive this vulnerable information sensitively and protect my heart. I needed their prayers as I tried to process what the heck this meant.

What Does it All Mean?

Let's define some terms to put this into context. A woman is officially considered to have entered "the menopause" when she goes one full year without having any bleeding. There are certain indications of perimenopause, for example: reaching age forty, having irregular cycles, hot flashes, and a blood test that confirms high FSH and low estrogen. A woman can be pre-menopause for years. It is possible to achieve pregnancy when in this category, but ovulation occurs less frequently. The average age of reaching menopause is fifty years old.

So, I started missing periods and not for the reason I wanted to be missing them, but I still had some hardcore hope. I thought, "all I need is one ovulation. God can do anything." There was no official confirmation that I was pre-menopausal, *yet*. You might have called that some shade of denial. Confirmation would have to come from FSH and estrogen labs. As I chewed on all this new information, I was also preparing for my one year post-operative visit with my NaPro surgeon in Houston after my eleventh surgery took place. The good news was that because I was having fewer periods, I was also having less pain, and this would please both myself and my surgeon.

I got my labs drawn right before our road trip to Texas. We combined this little "adventure" with a continuing education class Chris signed up for, also in Houston, and planned to visit his sister's family in Northwestern Louisiana on our way home. His other sister would bring Bella to meet us there, so I would have some free time to work on a very special new project.

Potential early grandma status was not the only "exciting" news I got prior to our trip. A local priest and all-star-modern-day-evangelist-for-all-ages friend of ours who refers to himself as "Funkie Fresh" invited me to re-write the sex and NFP chapter in a book he wrote for his engaged couples. It was a profound honor to be included in this incredibly creative educational tool which combines Church teaching, real life experiences, challenges, conversational questions, and an interactive component that allows the reader couples to receive videos and music that correspond to each chapter.

The purpose of this trek would be fourfold:
- Doc appointment
- Continuing ed class
- Visit Aunt Kim and family
- Rewrite chapter for priest friend

I dropped Chris off at class each morning and went back to the hotel room to pray and get to work. I was ecstatic to have about two full days to devote to the construction of this stellar chapter, which I hoped would describe God's amazing plan for sex, marriage, and fertility awareness in a way that was fresh, meaningful, interesting, and truly connecting with the target audience. This opportunity came at a time when I was in need of such a rejuvenation. It brought me to life!

You see, my purpose was expanding. What had started out as a ministry to help educate women of all ages about their health and fertility awareness options was transforming into a fuller mission of delivering the wonderful news about God's beautiful design of man and woman, *and* how that informs his plan for love and marriage. I had learned so much from being open and praying through our own experiences and I was thrilled to share that with others. God illuminated multiple perspectives for me that I knew would bring freedom to couples of all ages.

Hours flew by as I poured my heart and knowledge onto the pages (is my nerd showing again?) in hopes of educating, enlightening, and empowering prospective minds about the two primary purposes of sex, the challenges and beauty of marriage, and, of course, birth control and IVF explained, with alternatives included, and the health benefits of NFP/fertility awareness that are often left out of the conversation. There is a thirst for this information everywhere, but especially in marriage preparation. It was precisely my life journey up to that point, with all of its highs and incredibly low lows, that provided me with everything I needed to write that chapter and awaken new passions inside of me.

Writing had begun to take on a new life for me, and my blossoming mission wasn't far behind. And even as I anticipated what would likely be a very difficult meeting with my surgeon, I pondered and basked in the incredible joy my experience as a whole was bringing me. I armored up in prayer and threw on my favorite Blessed-Mother blue T-shirt that was perfect for the occasion, declaring, "She is clothed in strength and dignity (Proverbs 31:25)." This Bible chapter is rich. It paints the picture of *"a wife of noble character...who is worth far more than rubies"* (Proverbs 31: 10-11). She is hard working, a provider, selfless, resourceful, and prepared for anything; so much so, that "...*she can laugh at the days to come...*" It was the spirit of this woman described on my shirt that I hoped to walk into his office with.

11 Stripes

I arrived at my appointment alone because Chris was in class. That was rough, but sometimes it's helpful to process big news by yourself. I sank into his office chair donning my empowering threads draped with a Kelly-green cardigan and waited. He entered the room with his usual jovial smile, always making me feel welcome. I updated him on my recent doctor visit, told him about the hot flashes, and showed him my chart, hoping to get a different prognosis. Instead, I watched his face slowly droop into an expression you might recognize if you've ever told someone your dog just died. That face told me everything I needed to know.

The chart suggested perimenopause, but what really tipped him off was the occurrence of hot flashes in the absence of any medication. He then went on to explain some very important memos I had missed over the years. Multiple surgeries on the ovaries ("fertile" ground for endometriosis) *evidently* increase one's chances of early menopause. And I sat across from him with nearly eleven stripes against me in that department.

Regardless, all the surgeries were necessary. It was becoming clear that this menopause train was headed my way and there was nothing I could do to stop it. Time to achieve pregnancy was running out, but on the bright side, maybe this would spare me from a hysterectomy.

We headed to meet Bella and right before we pulled into Kim's driveway, I received a message from Dr. Caldwell's office with my lab results, which made the news official. I put my phone down and blankly stared out the car window as tears rolled down my cheeks and dripped right onto my lap.

Chris's sister lives on a lake in the country. There is plenty of open-spaced land and exquisitely framed views, perfect for gazing off into the sunset to contemplate life. Even though the door was only closing, it felt like it was already fully shut. Still, I could not help but feel so much hope and joy in anticipation of all God was doing in my life. That cathartic cry was my first and last on the subject. I made sure to feel the pain of my prognosis and continue to process all that it meant, but I was also prepared to move forward, keeping pace with the momentum at which God was unleashing me.

God positioned me appropriately to receive this news sensitively, feel its pain, and rejoice in it being part of a greater purpose. Although there were moments of shock, I received the first subtle clue when hot flashes interrupted my presentation. This prepared me for that local doctor visit. She didn't officially confirm anything, but spoke the words out loud that my heart needed to hear so it could begin to prepare itself. I got my blood drawn and ventured to Texas with the attitude and determination of a warrior headed into battle and determined to fight. I did not wait on the sidelines for a death sentence. God gave me important work to do that would fill my cup and inspire me with the promise of something beautiful that would continue to grow. He gave me something to look forward to. I didn't get the "yes" I was hoping for, but I dealt with it and continue to deal with every jarring reminder of reality. I allow myself to experience the hurt that is indicative of the loss of something intensely treasured. And I set my eyes on making beauty rise from ashes.

I could blame God for allowing my fertility to slowly take its final bow before using it to create a new life. I could fuss at Him for not ripping the bandaid off by telling me sooner. I could curse Him for giving me this dreaded uterus and ovaries in the first place. But how can I not be grateful for the woman He is shaping me into? How can I not be grateful that it brought us our adopted daughter? How can I not be grateful for awakening desires I had no idea were buried deep within my heart? It may be a different process for someone else, but the delicate delivery of this bad news over time was exactly what this girl needed. It is comforting to me to witness how intentional and tailor-made God's plans are. None of us are forgotten or slip through the cracks.

I had my meltdown moment, but I had so much to look forward to. No, I wasn't pregnant, and it didn't look like that was going to change any time soon, but I felt so alive! Still, if you can imagine, there were even more challenges to come.

CHAPTER 15

The Farewell Tour

"Faith is one foot on the ground, one foot in the air, and a queasy feeling in the stomach."
– *Mother Angelica*

As you can imagine, Mother's Day is one of the hardest days of the year for many infertile women. As time has passed and I have become inherently more fulfilled by what God has actually called me to, this infamous day has become less dreadful. I no longer approach it in fear or hide myself in the back rows of church just in case I burst out into tears or need to make a quick escape out the back door.

As my perspective on motherhood and infertility has become more enlightened, I have wanted to shout it from the rooftops––which is one of the many reasons why I have an Instagram account. As this past Mother's Day was approaching, I teamed up with my good friends Emily @totalwhine and Julianne @julianne_mcacy for a giveaway devoted to uplifting women by highlighting the beauty of spiritual motherhood in each individual person. The goal was to get women thinking about the numerous different ways they, *and* the people they love, grow new life into the world outside of the wonderful job of parenting little ones.

Julianne is one of my very best friends who has supported me and encouraged me to use my gifts since day one. We first became partners in crime back in high school when we were active in the same youth group and discovered that we have the same sense of humor. We have crafted the most ridiculous videos for our youth group and bachelorette friends––the latter, of course, had to include a couple of our favorite rap songs. She is one of few friends who shares a soft spot for a good beat with me. You can easily find us on a dance floor walkin' it out or joking about something outrageous. There is no one who can make me laugh like she does.

Her friendship has been priceless. She is also an incredibly gifted artist who has a particular fondness for the imagery of flowers. Luke 12:27 (NABRE) is her favorite Bible verse and is credited as the source of her inspiration: *"²⁷ Notice how the flowers grow. They do not toil or spin. But I tell you, not even Solomon in all his splendor was dressed like one of them."* Our giveaway needed to include one of her beautiful watercolor flowers, but which one? Julianne did some digging and found the most perfect symbol of suffering and growth. The Lotus.

She texted me in awe of the description she had just found: "Out of the murky mud of life grows the purely beautiful lotus flower, trusting in its own unfolding" (cardthartic.com). Evidently, lotus flowers are alluring aquatic plants, also referred to as water lilies, ranging in color from white to pink to purple and known for growing into these beauties from the murkiest of waters. Julianne draped a pinkish purple Lotus onto the thick textured paper and I hand lettered "Still Fruitful" beneath its roots.

This concept of the lotus flower provided me with the imagery I would be in great need of over the next several months and years. A mere five months prior to that Mother's Day was a New Year's Eve I'll never forget. A mid-December day, on which I was speaking to Dominican High School juniors about fertility awareness and Theology of the Body, brought an ovulation that triggered a resurgence of pain that I hadn't ever seen the likes of outside of my period. I popped the appropriate pain medication into my mouth, prayed hard to make it through my presentation, and breathed a sigh of relief when I arrived home safely. Like any other day of severe pain, I crawled into a warm bath, then settled into bed with my heating pad for the night expecting to feel fine the next morning. But I did *not* feel fine the next morning.

The discomfort confined me to my home and drastically limited my activity for weeks. It improved in intensity, giving me the ability to lie down or sit up and remain relatively comfortable, but I had trouble bending, walking, and lifting. I could no longer take on any speaking engagements because this pain proved to be so unpredictable. I was unable to care for Bella well, so her grandparents gave us some assistance. It was heartbreaking not to be able to care for my own child for such a long period of time. I could only imagine what my next period would bring, and it had its eye set on New Year's Eve.

We went to a friend's house to pop fireworks and ring in the new year. I spotted a chair that looked suitable for resting and got cozy for a couple of hours until I felt the pain begin to make its presence known. It's a classic feeling that is instantaneously recognizable—like a tap on the shoulder that I don't even need to turn in question of because I know exactly what's there. I gave Chris the signal and he took us home where the typical routine sprang into action.

I rested a while until midnight approached. He helped me walk out onto our backyard balcony for the countdown and to watch the fireworks dance over the trees in the distance. We took note and slow-danced for a while as we enjoyed the view. Chris helped to hold me up so we could remain close. I wrapped my arms tightly around him as tears erupted from my eyes in raging acknowledgment that this would be my last year with a physical womb.

Clean Up on Aisle Four

I was eleven surgeries deep at this point, spanning over a period of eight years. I was having two to three operations every two years. The pain was obviously returning and it would not have been right to continue to put Bella and my family through this roller coaster ride of recoveries and unpredictable pain just to keep my hope of bearing a child alive. I imagine this must sound crazy to many who are aware of the amount of physical pain I endured over the years. Yes, I agree that the natural response would be to "please remove this prickly death monster organ, and do it yesterday." But my womb didn't feel like *just* an organ, and it wasn't, even as prickly as it was. It is the body part that God provides every woman with to physically nurture and protect the miracle of every single human life. It is priceless. And in as much as I feared the cyclic pain, I had become strangely comfortable with it––preferring to experience that and the closeness it brought me with Jesus over parting with it, along with the aspiration of pregnancy. But at this point, clinging to that would have been selfish considering my long-term health and all the other people who would continue to be affected.

Because I "fought" so hard for so long, serious consideration of a hysterectomy felt like I had failed or was giving up and raising the white flag. I couldn't stand that imagery! But God showed me that it takes great strength to know when to stop and rest. It was not an acknowledgement of defeat, but bold acceptance of an invitation to shift the focus of my fight to something else—something I was born to do. I can't care for my daughter and family if I am unhealthy, nor can I go out into the world and complete the tasks I feel ardently called to.

It's not giving up or acknowledging defeat, but acknowledging reality. According to a reflection from Don Schwager, "True humility is not feeling bad about yourself, or having a low opinion of yourself...true humility frees us from preoccupation with ourselves...Humility is truth in self-understanding and truth in action. Viewing ourselves honestly, with sober judgement, means seeing ourselves the way God sees us (Psalm 139:1-4)."

It was time to begin preparing my heart for a new kind of break up.

I didn't realize it at the time, but God had been slowly preparing me for this all along. I know we hear it all the time in homilies and other talks, but I now know it to be true. Looking back on all of my long and drawn-out experiences, it has become evident that God is *always* ten steps ahead of each curveball with a much better plan already in place. Nothing catches him off guard. We are the ones that get ourselves knocked around like pinballs because we are so dyed in the wool for our own plans, which, pardon my language, but they suck. Trusting God in every individual day is flat out hard and it's something we typically learn how to do better *after* we fail at it a couple hundred thousand times.

My transformed, but always growing, outlook on life has blossomed from many failures. Another way to view challenges is as formation. My eight year journey through eleven surgeries is one avenue of many that has provided me with ample opportunities to fail and be formed. But you might read "eleven" surgeries and wonder how the heck they racked up.

Let me explain how I got here and how God has prepared me.

The One that Made it Worse
If you recall my first surgery, it was a #majorfail and required a second one to be scheduled only three months later. I was fortunate to keep my fertile organs the first time, but it was unlikely I would've been so lucky the second time around with my original doctor. I received the "okay" from my new NaPro doc in Nebraska and canceled operation number two in the nick of time.

With the extent of the disease's progression, which was unknown to me prior to surgery, and the promise of my doctor to be even more aggressive for round two, removal of crucial fertility organs was a thief lurking around the corner. Had I not been spared, unmarried at twenty-five years old, and without ever having the opportunity to even try to get pregnant and only several months after learning that I even had a disease in the first place, I would have gone into a surgery which I understood to be minimal and awakened to the shocking news that I was unable to bear children.

This was a great act of God's mercy. I would have been devastated had my hopes of getting pregnant been pulled out from under me so unexpectedly without getting the chance to try other treatments, discover suffering's purposes, unleash my gift of spiritual motherhood, and mentally and emotionally wrap my head around all of it.

The One that Gave me a C-Section Scar

There's something important to understand about the NaProTechnology approach to this type of surgery. As I'm sure you can imagine, the damage caused by endometriosis can be vast and extremely complicated. The only way to learn the extent of such is to go in surgically and take a thorough look around because ultrasounds and MRIs can only provide so much information.

So, they've coined a term called "first-look lap (laparoscopy)," which describes a minimally invasive diagnostic procedure where the doctor makes three small holes in the lower abdomen to insert a camera and other necessary instruments. If the damage is minimal, they'll correct it at that time. If they find that it's not so minimal, they'll use the video and pictures taken, study them, construct a comprehensive game plan, and come back well-prepared to tackle the effects of the disease during a second procedure.

I have had four "first look laps", which is part of the reason I've racked up so many surgeries. It was my inaugural one that called for my first flight to Omaha, Nebraska, and it took place about seven months after my first surgery and revealed how extensive the spread of the disease was, as well as that dadgum scar tissue. It, without question, required a second surgery that would be major in nature. At the time, my physicians had not yet mastered the not-so-invasive techniques of the Davinci Robot, so this meant I needed a laparotomy––a word which still makes me cringe at its sight because it required such a long and painful recovery.

This was my third surgery that took place two days after Chris popped the question, lasted about six and a half hours, and gave me a six inch scar a few inches below my belly button. She removed my appendix which was riddled with disease, that ten centimeter endometrioma, scar tissue, endometriosis, and/or fibroids in a total of sixteen other locations. Yea––sixteen.

The One that Caused me to Switch Doctors, Again
Let me tell you a little something about scar tissue, which is best described as that annoying jerk who tags along to a party with the other uninvited house guests. "Adhesions" are bands of scar tissue and can be caused by both the disease *and* surgery. Scar tissue is known to cause pain and infertility in and of itself and is a known risk factor heading into any operation. It is also well-supported that individuals produce scar tissue differently, so you don't know how your body will respond until it happens. I had a decent amount of experience with this as a Physical Therapist Assistant who treated many post-operative knee and shoulder replacements, as well as ACL and rotator cuff repairs for six years. I was entrusted with the task of stretching these men and women's joints in an effort to prevent scar tissue from forming, and even break through it to maintain and/or improve range of motion. You've heard the term "physical terrorists?" I was one of em'! Scar tissue affects each person differently depending on the individual *and* the part of the body where the surgery occurs.

This brings us to another unique and very special aspect of NaProTechnology surgeries that is important to understand, but may also blow your mind. The Journal of Gynecologic Surgery published research conducted by Dr. Thomas Hilgers entitled, "Near Adhesion-Free Reconstructive Pelvic Surgery: Three Distinct Phases of Progress Over 23 Years[12]." *Yes, twenty-three years!* In the abstract, Hilgers basically explains that some physicians shy away from surgery due to potential adhesions to be formed, which is associated with long-term morbidity. But endometriosis is a surgical disease and there's no getting around that. So, he developed a surgical technique which allows NaPro-trained surgeons to help even the most severely affected patients, but with a drastically improved "near-adhesion-free" outcome. He was able to reduce total adhesion scores from 33.2 to 2.5!

There are many fascinating components of his groundbreaking technique. One of them is called a "second-look laparoscopy," which was devised in response to the understanding that the majority of scar tissue forms within eight to ten days after major surgery. If a much more minimally invasive procedure is conducted to simply remove as much of that scar tissue as possible, it will reduce long-term occurrence. I have had two "second-look laps."

Another fascinating detail is the use of an "adhesion barrier," which we always referred to as "gortex." This is a uniquely developed material used to "pack away" all fertile organs applicable in order to protect them from adherence to other organs like the bowel. Scar tissue becomes a sort of glue which causes pain and infertility by joining organs together that are supposed to be free and docile. There is either a large or small gortex used in these surgeries, depending on the area affected. The smaller one can actually remain permanently, but the larger one is removed along with any scar tissue present during the second-look lap.

During my laparotomy, which was extensive, my physician made a judgement call to use the smaller gortex when she should've used the larger one. It turned out that I, unfortunately, am one of those individuals who produces a vast amount of scar tissue. As a result, the gortex got tangled up with my left ovary and associated scar tissue that formed in excess of her expectations and required another surgery years later.

My endometriosis had been managed pretty well this time. It did recur, but at a much improved rate with appropriate surgical management. It was the scar tissue that my body had been rapidly producing that has caused one of a few additional problems. We really liked my second doctor, but as we continued to learn how complicated my situation was, and with the results of her judgement call, we decided to switch to another NaPro doctor who had more experience.

The One Where It Opened Like a Flower

As my abdominal cavity had its eyes set on round three of surgeries, a significant amount of unusual bleeding began to pop up on my Creighton chart. Remember, this charting system is uniquely used to gain important information about what's going on inside of the woman's body. In this case, it was possible that the bleeding was being caused by another new fancy six syllable word I was about to learn: a-den-o-my-o-sis.

I like to refer to adenomyosis as endometriosis' meaner, uglier, and nastier stepsister. Endometriosis implants on the surface of organs. The "stepsister" burrows itself into the actual wall of the uterus. It tends to grow with spider-like veins throughout, so the only treatment is to remove the muscle of the uterus. My new doctor alerted me to the existence of this other women's health disease that could have been causing much of my relentless pain and the unusual bleeding.

This was the first time "hysterectomy" was thrown out as a potential treatment plan. He wasn't recommending it presently, but explaining it as the only treatment for a progressive disease I may have. This struck me in a moderately terrifying way as I felt my clock instantly speed up. You know how the good guy tries to disarm a bomb in the movies and cuts the wrong wire first, which causes the time to begin ticking faster?

That's what was happening in my mind.

It's worth mentioning that a hysterectomy will "cure" adenomyosis (because that can only be located within the uterus), but it won't cure endometriosis. As long as an ovary is present, endometriosis can be produced and spread, so it is important that the surgeon removing the uterus does his or her best to eliminate any endometriosis present at the time of surgery. No one was signing me up for the ultimate fertility death blow, but even the suggestion of such made me quiver. He would get a better look at the situation during my next operation, where I would meet Dr. Stephen Hilgers, the son of the great mind behind NaProTechnology.

Dr. Stephen Hilgers introduced himself to Chris and I during the pre-op of this fifth operation. At the time, he was one of the Fellows training to learn these classic NaProTechnology surgical techniques in Nebraska. The St. Pope Paul VI Institute offers a specialized year-long process that OB/GYNs can go through in addition to their medical school training and provide to their own patients anywhere in the world. Dr. Stephen was one of the doctors who would be present during my next surgery. We met a new Fellow every time we visited Omaha.

Physicians in surgery number five ended up removing that small gortex that was left behind during surgery number three, but they also reconstructed my left ovary and tube which had been pretty badly mangled. Dr. Stephen explained to me how beautifully the fimbria at the end of the fallopian tube "opened like a flower" after they spent hours working at it meticulously. Let me just tell you––these are the types of doctors you want fighting for your fertility in the operating room. A fibroid attached to my uterus was also biopsied and confirmed the presence of adenomyosis, but nothing further was mentioned about it at that time.

By the time this operation arrived, my doctors had mastered the Da Vinci Surgical System, which is an incredible advancement in technology which allows the surgeon to control the five tiny hands of a robot with far more range of motion and dexterity than a human. The doctor is seated several feet away from the patient and uses a video and controls, kind of like a video game, and allows them to accomplish many of the incredible tasks of an open surgery but by using a much less invasive procedure with only five holes. This grants a much improved recovery for the patient.

The One that Made Him Say "Whoops"

About two more years passed and my pain began to increase. Again. I know, it's exhausting to even read this scenario. I still wasn't pregnant. I also had a new complication associated with my cycles to add to the list: rectal pain. And it was getting worse. We headed back to Omaha to begin my next round of first-look lap, robotic surgery, then second-look lap. A colo-rectal surgeon made himself available this time around in case he would be needed to perform surgery on my bowel. He ended up not being used. It became clear that my left ovary had not healed as nicely as expected and was not releasing an egg consistently, if at all.

Because the average woman typically alternates between ovaries when ovulating every month, I figured that this was hurting my chances of conceiving. I asked my doctor what he thought about removing the left ovary so that I could hopefully ovulate out of the right ovary every cycle, making pregnancy more likely. He was receptive to this idea.

I recognize that this may sound unusual considering what I went through to keep all my fertile organs. But by now, we had years of trying to achieve pregnancy under our belt and it still wasn't happening. Also, as long as you have an ovary, it can produce endometriosis and endometriomas. I believed that keeping my left ovary intact at this point was doing more harm than good. It was a sad day, but I felt confident that we were making the right decision, and he removed it.

This is when things got interesting. A couple more years passed and pain during my periods increased exponentially this time––like nothing I had ever experienced. I later discovered that this occurred for three reasons, one of which I'll explain now. I had multiple ultrasounds and an MRI to help my local doctor understand what was causing the pain. They were unable to find anything extremely unusual, but they continued to tell me they identified my left ovary. I told them that this was impossible because I didn't have a left ovary. This "thing" that resembled an ovary would also appear in different locations. It was a true mystery. After it was finally biopsied, we learned that it was an endometrioma that had grown from a cellular piece of my ovary that was dropped in my abdomen upon its removal during a previous surgery.

Whoops.

Pretty spectacular, right? But, like, not in a good way.

The One with the Franken-uterus
As I just mentioned, the pain I began to deal with as my tenth and eleventh surgeries approached became something I could have never imagined. The first time

it hit me was a Saturday morning I'll never forget. I woke up and walked into my bathroom, but couldn't leave on my own accord. I needed an emergency room and I needed it five minutes ago. Chris carried me from the bathroom floor to the car and we barely escaped the driveway before I started to throw up in response to the pain.

The fifteen minute drive felt like hours. Once we arrived, I hobbled into the closest wheelchair, writhing and folded over, motioning for a vomit bag. I was too focused on surviving to feel embarrassed. I used that infamous blue handheld bag as I was rolled past the nurse's station and into one of the rooms.

The rest is a blur until the second dose of morphine kicked in. I remember frantically kicking my flip flops off as Chris helped the nurses to get me into a robe and to hold me down so they could draw blood and start an IV. It's hard to find a vein with so much movement. Later my sister arrived to my empty room (when they took me for an ultrasound) to find what she described as a crime scene with my flip flops and blood scattered on the floor from attempts to stick my vein. A catheter was needed to get a urine sample.

Then there was more waiting...

A nurse can't prescribe morphine and it takes time for the doctor to come. *And* they had to make sure I wasn't on drugs.

I remember rocking back and forth with eyes clenched, hands gripping the bed rails, and feet digging into those classic white sheets. My life wasn't in danger, but I remember wondering if I was going to die. I remember feeling guilty for hoping someone would knock me out of consciousness to get a moment of relief. "Where is the will to get through this? Find it, Mary..."

Finally, the morphine arrived. The nurse said it would make my whole body feel weird for a moment and then that would go away. She was right. On a normal day, that anticipation would've caused me great anxiety. But all I could think of was the potential relief it would bring.

As that magical fluid trickled through my veins for the second time (because one dose wasn't quite enough), my limbs finally began to relax into the bed and a sigh of relief exited my mouth with the next few breaths. Now able to appreciate the back of my eyelids, I rested perfectly still, and completely soaked up every ounce of that very simple feeling that we often take for granted: normalcy.

It was clearly time for another doctor appointment. And just to give you some insight into this complex women's health condition that so many females struggle with mentally just as much as they struggle with it physically––the only conclusion the ER medical team could give me was that my uterus had several fibroids. They sent me home with some pain medicine.

Now I set out to find more answers. I found out that after he finished his Fellowship, Dr. Stephen Hilgers set up a practice in Houston Methodist Hospital, which is much closer to my home in New Orleans than Nebraska. So, I made another switch and the Institute sent what probably felt like truckloads of medical records to my new doctor in Texas to review. He examined all information, which included my recent ultrasounds and MRI results, and scheduled a phone consult with me to discuss a plan.

In addition to the mysterious ovary-looking object (which hadn't yet been biopsied), he noticed an enlarged uterus–like, *really* enlarged–and suspected adenomyosis, that evil stepsister of endometriosis. Considering my history and present symptoms, he cautiously and gently uttered the words I had most feared hearing for years: "I think you're going to need a hysterectomy."

This time that word wasn't being used in a hypothetical "sometime in the distant future" way, but in an "I don't think you can wait any longer" way. When a NaPro surgeon makes that suggestion, you know it's serious because they don't use that term lightly.

I was only thirty-two years old. Time stopped for the third time in my life. I locked eyes with Chris from across the kitchen table where my phone sat, those heartbreaking words echoing through my mind. I asked the doctor if he would go in for the hysterectomy immediately, but he said he would feel more comfortable performing a first-look lap to get a well-formed picture of what was going on beneath the surface. The rest of the conversation was fuzzy. I hung up the phone and wept, asking Chris to give me a moment by myself.

The next several days passed in slow motion as I attempted to process this prognosis. I was confident that every surgery would be the last, but each series of operations would only give me about a two year breathing window and then we were back at it again. Whatever was growing inside of me was aggressive, and relentless. It was like a recurring nightmare. It made no sense to keep having surgeries unless something would be dramatically different.

I figured this final step would come eventually, but was hoping it would hold off until after we had a child or three. Even if I had given birth previously, what woman doesn't feel the deep and painful loss of her womb—the carrier of human life that is unique to woman alone? It appeared as though time had officially slipped away. This brought on more anger with the crippling sense of control crumbling beneath me and inspired the first verse of *"Choices:"*

I'm sore inside from dealing with this pain
And I'm tired of running with no ground to gain
Like dry ice in the theater thoughts are clouding my mind
They go from weak to bleak to miracles of all kinds
I'm workin' real hard to keep this boat afloat
Clingin' to every single syllable of hope
But I'm taking on water and slowly sinking
I'm all ears God if you wanna start speakin'
Gave you time and effort and good decisions
And you're payin' me back with this final revision?
Look I know. I've got my own big plans,
But this is personal. You don't understand.
I can't escape the pain, it's just too much
And you could take it away–with just one touch
Our wills collide, so I'm sittin on the fence.
I can't take any more of your loud silence...

I allowed myself to be honest about my anger, but I was also given the grace to recognize that these were "only" my feelings. And although they were very real and absolutely mattered, they were a reflection of thoughts that were not true. I didn't always *feel* it, but I knew how much God loved me; how much He cared. I knew my pain was hurting Him, too, and I decided to write the second verse of this song from His perspective and how I imagined He would respond:

I know too well of your bruised and your brokenness–
The feelings of betrayal from your heart's wide openness.
I know it 'cuz I made your weakness into My own
When you hurt, I hurt too–your pain is never alone
Although I hate to see you crying in the depths of your pain,
These are the very same depths that will ignite your flame.
The pavement's hard but it's a great place to start
Strike it with a match – I'm lightin' up the corners of your heart!
Living fulfilled isn't gonna be easy.
But you make the choice–who you gonna be pleasing?
Put your fingers in My side and feel the pulse in My veins.
This love is real like your decision. Take the reins!
I'm just a breath away–I'll wait as long as it takes.
You can't push me away–even with your mistakes.
You don't have to look far when you're searching for guidance.
But you had it right first. Find Me in the silence!
Hook:
I'm driving down a road to an uncertain future
Tugging on my wounds; pulling out my sutures
My scars are deep, but they're telling my story
It's up to me if it's gory or glory

This song became another cathartic release for me. I connect with it because it marries bitter honesty with loving compassion and the choice we all have the opportunity to make towards healing. The result gives hope and is expressed in the conclusion of the final verse: "I've got to look North to find my Perfection. What could have been my death just became my resurrection." It helped me to find the will to press on. I pondered that dreaded *hysterectomy* word in disbelief, kept His comforting presence close to my heart, and moved forward one step at a time.

I made a conscious effort to mourn and experience this deep grief, but not without an openness to Christ moving inside of me. I cannot fully explain what I experienced next, even within my expression of deep sorrow, other than by describing the presence of a profound and steady grace from God that fostered true acceptance. There is something incredibly freeing about the willful acceptance of God and His will when we are able to disconnect from our personal preferences. It is not a promise to remove grief, but makes ample room for His healing presence and hope for tomorrow. I was somehow able to offer my fertility as a gift to God to do with as He pleases.

I had a few months to prepare myself for the next operation which would direct my doctor's plan for my final surgery, but my post-operative visit ended up delivering a pretty big surprise. After peering directly into my abdominal cavity, Dr. Stephen Hilgers came back to Chris and I and depicted my enlarged uterus as a "Franken-uterus." He actually made up a word to describe it which made us laugh out loud. Three large adenomyomas (cysts of adenomyosis) had formed into the base of my uterus, making it two times the size of a normal one. This was, no doubt, largely contributing to my agony. He also found that my bowel was largely scarred over and would demand a colo-rectal surgeon's expertise, ultimately requiring a bowel resection. And there was also that endometrioma sitting at the bottom of my abdominal cavity.

My new Texas doctor was shocked at what he witnessed inside of me and continued to amaze by adding an intriguing option for Chris and I to ponder before moving forward. One choice would clearly be to go ahead and remove the uterus. There's nothing fascinating about that. But because, fortunately, most of the adenomyosis was localized, he gave us the opportunity to have the bottom portion of my enlarged uterus cut off (myomectomy) then sewed back together, keeping the possibility of pregnancy intact! I was stunned. This would require a C-section if we would ever be able to conceive, but heck, who am I to complain if it means I get to keep my uterus *and* have a baby? I'd be pulling out the confetti again! He gave Chris and I a few days to think and pray about our decision.

We both went into the procedure assuming it would deem that a hysterectomy was necessary. But this first look lap gave us three pieces of brand new information which kept our hope of conceiving, and simply holding onto all my organs, alive. I would not have felt comfortable enduring a full removal without exhausting every possible option. I would have always wondered what might have happened, so we scheduled the myomectomy.

My eleventh surgery was another long one which provided for the removal of that mysterious endometrioma, about a third of my uterus, and about six to eight inches of bowel, three days before Easter. On my operative day, I walked into the hospital feeling literally weighed down by the disease and scar tissue that insisted on attacking my insides. I woke up from surgery and instantly felt that weight completely lifted. Surgeries in the past had improved my pain, but this was the first one that eliminated it. It was the first one that enforced the eviction notice given to my adenomyosis.

I prepared for my first period after surgery with over the counter anti-inflammatories just as a precaution, but felt almost no pain. It was an unreal experience compared to a month prior where prescription strength anti-inflammatories, narcotics, and daily nerve-pain medicine couldn't control it. Only morphine. I even had a dramatic reduction in the heaviness of my bleeding. For the first time as a woman with a period, I experienced what I imagined to be "normal."

I didn't know what to do with myself. I could make plans and go out into public like a normal person—even during Aunt Flow's visits! Is this how normal women function? Regardless of what was going to happen next, it was a real privilege to be able to live some perception of normalcy as a young woman. I was even able to hope for pregnancy again, seeing as everything seemed to have been repaired better than ever before. My uterus lived to see another day, and I was cautiously optimistic.

I continued to breathe a sigh of relief, but although my pain had greatly improved, my cycle never really got the message that things had been fixed. My body had been through a lot. My hormones never stabilized and my body hardly responded to the bio-identical supplementation that had worked in the past. It wasn't consistent with every cycle, but several months later delivered a brand new painful period. Several months after that, and during my second week of training to become a Creighton Practitioner, brought one that was even more uncomfortable. How ironic? As I prepared to advance my knowledge and understanding of health and fertility to help other women, my own insides were being attacked by itself. This made training extremely difficult, but I made it through by the grace of God and the wonderful support of my classmates and supervisor.

Not long afterwards, I learned that my cycles began to resemble pre-menopause as the result of so many surgeries on my ovaries. A visit to Dr. Stephen Hilgers and a local blood draw confirmed it as I entered into "hot mess" territory. It was a shocking new reality, but gave us hope that I would be able to keep my uterus intact since periods would become fewer and more far in between until eventually stopping permanently, along with the pain.

It became a race to the finish line–which would tire out first? Would it be my ovaries or my uterus? My ovaries began to shut down, but could still have years of life left even if not to full capacity. The case for my womb didn't appear to be so strong as it began to make a glaringly obvious plea to be put out of its misery. I could only deny its request for so long. Each surgery had me unknowingly participating in the farewell tour of my fertility, but I thank God that that is how it happened.

I could be bitter about Him not putting me out of my misery sooner, which would have allowed me to avoid so many painful and costly surgeries, travel, menstrual cycles, and heartache. Maybe that would've served someone else better, but God's plans are tailor-made. I have experienced depth of life, growth, and healing *because of* the very sufferings I have lived through–*not* despite them. Each knock stretched and molded me into the person I am today. I can look back in awe of what Christ has worked with me to overcome with immense gratitude, but the work is never done. I could have never anticipated how I was about to react to the newer depths of Christ's heart I was about to venture into.

CHAPTER 16

The Twelfth Stripe

"Faith is what gets you started. Hope is what keeps you going. Love is what brings you to the end."
— Mother Angelica

I WAS IN AN INTIMATE PRAYER group with four other Catholic women a few years ago. In one of our book studies, my eyes were opened to a concept that was simple, but riveting, "Consoling the Heart of Jesus[13]." In this book, Fr. Michael Gaitley describes a deep longing within Jesus Himself: *"Behold this Heart which loves so much yet is so little loved. Is there anyone who will console this Heart? Is there anyone who will be my friend?"* St. Therese of Lisieux adds to this in her encounter of the humanity of the Eucharistic Heart of Jesus. *"She sees a man who has feelings, a man who is hurt when people are cold, ungrateful, and afraid of Him.[13]"* She enlightens us further to a desire to console His heart, which feels so neglected.

Initially, it's easy to think that the physical agony of His crucifixion would be the source of His most intense pain. But Gaitley insists that Jesus' heart burns with such extraordinary love for us in His longing to forgive. Accepting His mercy quenches the flames a bit and consoles His heart, but many souls don't seek His forgiveness. "Jesus sees humanity's pain constantly–in every detail–and it shatters His heart. Thus, Jesus desperately longs to reach out with His saving, healing, and consoling touch. Whether or not He can, depends in large part on us."

There are a few different things we can take from this reflection. One point reminds us that Jesus is fully Divine, but is also fully human. He understands the longings and desires of the human heart well because He has experienced all of them. He knows quite well what it means to feel forgotten. Another important and comforting point of contemplation lends to a better understanding of how desperately Christ desires to ease our own pain––so much so, that His heart doesn't rest until ours do. He is just as invested in the purity and peace of our hearts as we are––even more so. It often seems like

He is working against us when things don't go as we have planned because we are aware that God can make anything happen with the snap of a finger. But He is not a magician. He is a lover. And a lover considers what is best for His beloved and makes those desires His own.

On my worst day ever, I did not feel like His beloved. But as I recall those days with a reflective heart that has accepted His invitation to go deeper, I can see more clearly. I can see a Lover who is patient and who will spare no expense to reach my heart. Oh, the pain I must have caused Him when I looked at Him with blame! Oh, how it must have hurt Him to refuse me the comfort I sought to have me choose Himself no matter what! There was only one thing he desired greater than consoling my heart at that moment in time, and that was winning my heart outright to award Him the pleasure of consoling it for an eternity.

I am so grateful He has prevailed in His unfailing pursuit of me because He has equipped me for other trials to come. That New Year's Eve moment that provoked a realization of my impending final surgery took place almost two years after my myomectomy, a time period which had become all too familiar. Within the next two weeks, my hysterectomy was scheduled. There would be no first look lap to give any wiggle room for escaping my fate this time. Settling on an official date made it real and kicked off the official countdown towards the very last days of possible fertility. Fortunately, I had a couple of months to prepare my heart.

Days and weeks passed. I made sure to go into the deep crevices of my heart to make sure I was appropriately dealing with what was about to happen. I made a conscious effort to be honest about all my *thoughts* and *feelings* because I know from experience what happens when those aren't addressed. I prayed hard and focused on gratitude. I didn't want any lies to creep in and confuse me about my identity as a woman and daughter of God, or recognition of my motherhood.

I had never devoted so much valuable time and attention to my spiritual and emotional health, an effort which, joined with the years God invested into this preparation, produced the most stunning fruit. Many will consider eleven surgeries to be overkill. I view it as a great mercy because my heart made great use of that time, and I needed to know that absolutely everything had been tried before agreeing to the last resort. That date continued to creep closer, but my peace only grew. My joy was only enhanced. There is no earthly explanation for the profound comfort I experienced daily, even in the face of great sadness.

What a juxtaposition this was when stacked against my worst day ever! It was in direct contrast to the comfort I sought after learning of my false positive pregnancy test. My bitterness was magnified by a repetitive denial of *my* plans and *my* perception of both womanhood and motherhood. But God didn't give up on me. He broke through my walls and with my permission, took this broken woman with a broken uterus and transformed her into someone with great purpose who not only understands, but values herself for exactly who she is and how she was made. Even standing before the crystal-clear recognition of permanent infertility, I was okay. I was sad, but I was okay. There was no blame. I didn't need to ask for comfort because he was already lavishing it upon me.

It was strange to be so at peace during this time. I was uncharacteristically joyful, but I couldn't complain about that. On the contrary, I desired nothing more than to share this account of hope, which ended up coming together in a very unexpected way. I did not set out to write this book. As a long-time blogger, it seemed fitting to create a series of posts describing this story which carried me through so many hills and valleys, and ultimately great hope. I wrote three blog posts which eventually became chapters one, five, and seven as the Holy Spirit unleashed Himself onto many pages, revealing what would soon unfold into the book you presently hold in your hands. The lies I believed about a prescribed form of living out my faith as a Catholic woman were replaced with the magnificent truth. Despite the inability to procreate, God was not done with me. Who says I need a uterus to bear fruit?

The One that Took my Uterus
I enjoyed the unexplainable peace I graciously lived in, but kept waiting for the other shoe to drop. I imagined

myself packing for Houston by violently throwing clothes into my suitcase out of anger while soaking each shirt and set of pants with my tears. Would Chris have to carry me to the car? Surely I wasn't comprehending how real this was.

But when the time came, I packed up my bags and walked to the car just fine.

Then I imagined Chris having to carry me, bawling crying, out of the hotel to head to my pre-op room so they could prep me for surgery. Surely then it would feel real.

But when the time came, I left the room on my own accord just fine. I even snapped a cute picture of Chris and I walking down the street at five a.m.

Finally, I thought for sure they would have to pry my cold, dead fingers off of the door jam as they wheeled me out of that pre-op room and into the operating room.

But when the time came, they wheeled me without complaint. I did the hard internal work to prepare for this day. God was faithful to His promises.

Chris and I had arrived in Houston several days early to escape another hurricane that was headed toward Louisiana.

We ended up really enjoying what became a mini vacation—maybe a "hysterectomoon?"—in that big Texas town, sightseeing, taste testing at different restaurants, enjoying margaritas, visiting a fancy garden, and simply enjoying each other. You would've never known I was about to have the most dreaded surgery of my life.

On the eve of surgery, I had to fast because operating would require an empty stomach. Chris stepped out to grab a bite to eat, and this provided a few much-needed moments alone to pow-wow with my Maker. We stayed on floor twenty-something of a hotel with a huge bay window, which left us with a breathtaking view of the city. My gaze stretched miles deep, locking eyes with the setting sun, wrapped in yellow, and outstretching its orangy-red arms as if to embrace me. It was a stunning backdrop for my intimate moment with God. The colorful mix of clouds was a calming scene mimicking His peaceful influence on my heart. I cried. It was hard to believe that this long and hard-fought journey was ending and preparing the way for a new one to begin. Once again, I took the opportunity to thank God for all the gifts He has given me. I offered Him my pain and invited Him to make use of it as I said my final goodbyes to any hope of biological children. There was a death about to take place here, but there was also new life being formed all around me.

I have the love of a guy who sincerely cares for me at my worst and is equally as joyful about the prospects of our future, even though it was looking nothing like we had planned. When I was younger, I had my life figured out just like I had my future husband figured out, but God blew both of my ideas out of the water.

I not only had the sincere and devout love of two men, one on earth and One in heaven, but I felt it. How could I not be joyful?

This surgery marked the twelfth stripe on a long list of operations leaving a total of fourteen unique scars. Scar tissue, of course, through a few curve balls that were ultimately taken care of. My colon surgeon was back to do some cleanup work as well. And I had a surprise visit from a urologic surgeon.

Generally, as I come out of anesthesia, I slowly become more and more aware of my surroundings while my eyes remain closed. I hear nurses talking and typing information, asking me about my pain, to which I respond with vague grunts, and administering medication, etc. Then at some point, transportation comes and wheels my bed into the elevator (where I feel every bump), and into my recovery room. The nurse then helps him or her to not-so-cautiously transfer me onto the next hospital bed by using those classic white sheets. That part is always pretty uncomfortable. Like, do they not realize I just had major surgery?

This immediate post-op experience was no different than the other ones until the grogginess finally wore off and I opened my eyes. Previously, I had imagined that at this point, I would certainly wake from anesthesia and immediately burst into uncontrollable tears as I became more and more aware of where I was and what had just happened. But that didn't happen either.

As I emerged from my deep sleep, the first thing I saw was Chris's smiling face. The second thing I saw was a crisp, white lotus floating in dirty water hanging on the hospital room wall. This is the very plant that signifies growth from the most unexpected of environments, and that my friend Julianne drew for our giveaway. This 16x20 beauty was framed on the wall in perfect view and protected by crystal clear glass.

I instantly felt my heart hugged by Christ Himself. It was impossible for me to feel forgotten at this point as He made sure I knew how intensely treasured I was at the most perfect moment. The magnitude of this surgery, its permanence, and the invitation into my heart was not lost on Him. Right away, He provided a meaningful reminder that the loss of my uterus said nothing about the beauty He will continue to bring into the world through the murky waters of my life. I will always be limited by my human nature, but Christ within me cannot be contained.

Several days later, we arrived home to begin recovery. I was still at peace. Chris and I also had a post-op phone consultation with Dr. Stephen Hilgers where he would assess my recovery and discuss some surgery details. He expressed that the amount of disease I had developed over the years was quite impressive, noting that he even found endometriosis within my fallopian tube––which occurs in only fourteen percent of pre-menopausal women according to research in the *Journal of Minimally Invasive Gynecology*[14] and is extremely difficult to diagnose.

This certainly added another layer to reasons why pregnancy couldn't have occurred barring a miracle. Fortunately, Chris and I were at a place where we could laugh at how impossible pregnancy had actually become. It really seemed as though we may have never had a chance! This was strangely satisfying to me as I considered that God had always truly designed another path for us.

My friend, Elise, who helped me to discover and dive into my rapping genius, was unable to visit me due to the Coronavirus pandemic, so she mailed me a sweet card instead. As I opened the "Get well quick…" cover to a "…you're too nice to be sick" message, a hand-written note dropped on the floor. It had been written on my surgery day, and I want to share some of what she said:

"My sister,
...After praying and thanking God for keeping you safe...it hit me like a ton of bricks! Your uterus is gone. I couldn't stop crying. I hesitated to even write this, but then God put it on my heart that you need to know that someone mourned for your loss today. It wasn't just me but what He was allowing me to feel the great sadness that He was feeling for your loss and your pain! He recognizes your sacrifice for Him, your strength, your courage, your intense perseverance!...He recognizes your surrender to His will and He is overcome with joy that you continue to choose Him!

...I know that if this is His plan...then literally today is the birth of something new! I cannot wait to see what true fertility God has in store for your life. He is releasing you of the weight of not knowing and calling you from physical pain...to be reborn and be created new because...He has so much work for you to do...nothing can hold you back now..."

The words on the paper struck my heart immediately, instantly calling to mind Fr. Michael Gaitley and company's thoughts on "Consoling the heart of Jesus.[13]" Even as Christ's heart burns due to lack of care and attention given by so much of humanity, He longs to embrace my own little heart with His comforting presence and make my suffering His own. He longed for me to know that He mourned the loss of something so significant and precious right along with me. *"Jesus sees humanity's pain constantly–in every detail–and it shatters His heart. Thus, Jesus desperately longs to reach out with His saving, healing, and consoling touch...[13]"*

Several days later, I received another generous and thoughtful gift from my other close friend, Lisa. I opened up a small gift box decorated with gold flowers to find a purple velvet pouch holding a small lotus flower charm dangling from a beautiful rose gold necklace.

Purpose Blossoms
Physical recovery took a bit longer than expected, so Chris, Bella, and I moved in with my parents for a couple of months. My mom's servant heart has sprung into action beautifully after each surgery and this time was no exception. She once again provided me with the much-needed rest required to get back to normal. It didn't take too long for my creativity, mission to empower women, and desire to write to come back online.

Ripe with emotion from surgery, I continued to develop this memoir and even began to formulate my book proposal. Putting the words of my experiences throughout the years down has been incredibly healing and has allowed me to feel even more purpose. It was also during this time that a nearly year-long collaborative project with two good friends, Emily @totalwhine and Jen @surprisedbymarriage, finally came together and was published. *"Uncharted Territory"* is a series of six written conversations struck up between the three of us combining raw, honest, and beautiful fertility awareness testimonies from our three completely different perspectives––infertile, fertile, and subfertile.

Our teamwork and common passions blossomed so beautifully over that year, that it inspired Emily and I to discern partnering up for a business venture that would allow us to dramatically improve fertility awareness education, access, and solidarity. God has allowed unique and painful experiences in both of our lives and equipped us with the personalities, abilities, and drive to be two of many who serve Him with this mission.

So, less than a month after surgery we theoretically broke ground on what would eventually become a 501(c)3 non-profit organization, called FAbM Base (pronounced FAM-base), of which I presently serve as Executive Director. Our website, www.fabmbase.org, exists to help women and couples to find the fertility awareness-based method that fits them best, educate women of all ages on birth control and alternatives to that and ART, help them to find restorative reproductive medicine, and provide a space where people who experience the various difficult and rarely discussed topics regarding NFP use can come together for support.

I do not think this timing was accidental. The end of an era of fertility problems and wavering hope was heartbreaking. But it also almost instantly breathed life into even greater opportunities for my life and sense of purpose. We also found a new adoption agency that we are much more comfortable with and are presently awaiting God to send Bella a brother or sister in His time. How can I not be joyful?

I understand that this is a book that largely describes a range of my personal experiences, fears, joys, and talents. It is cathartic, but it also feels very strange and oftentimes uncomfortable to talk about myself in this way. I am not hoping to simply tell you a story about myself. I hope to communicate the possibilities available by way of faith in Christ. They go well beyond our own imagination because God is not limited like we are. I want you to understand the immeasurable value in yourself *as you are,* and in being honest about how you feel in regards to the sufferings that God allows in this life. Grasp their potential use. It is easy to hold firm when our ground is not shaking, causing our world to fall apart. The true test of our faith occurs when the Richter Scale comes into play and tests the very foundation on which we stand.

It is possible to reach a place where hope *cannot* fail despite life's nastiest curveballs--when we believe in God's unfailing attention to our best interests.

Tested
Earlier this year, Bella went to her yearly checkup and failed her hearing test. It wasn't all that surprising because even though she speaks very well, she often has a hard time hearing us and the TV. The audiologist that fitted her for hearing aids recommended that we come back every six months instead of the typical yearly follow up to see if her hearing loss is progressive...to which we responded "progressive?!" We didn't even know that was a possibility. But because she passed her newborn hearing test, and had now failed multiple, it would be wise to check routinely.

Well, this certainly wasn't on our radar. My brain instinctively wanted to go down an imaginary rabbit hole of *what ifs*. What if this *is* progressive? What if she becomes completely deaf before she even becomes a teenager? What would that look like? How on earth would we operate? How will her peers treat her? Oh my goodness, the list could go on forever. But I caught myself after those first several depressing questions to offer myself another perspective in light of what my battle with infertility did for me.

Let's say she does completely lose her hearing. It would certainly be very scary for everyone, especially her, at first. She would miss that precious ability we all take for granted for probably the rest of her life. We would all need to mourn. But she would learn a plethora of new things. We would all get creative and figure out how to communicate. We would focus our attention on gratitude for what we do have and all we have learned through this experience. Yes, she would have trials, but she would also have the opportunity to become stronger from all of it. And who knows what other little girl or boy's life with similar struggles she would impact.

None of life's headaches or "inconvenient hotels," as my heavenly BFF (St. Teresa of Avila) so eloquently put it, are

shocking for our Creator. He has planned for every single one of them. We humanize God when we blame or forget Him when things don't go our way, as if we are being ignored or are less important than our neighbor, whose life appears to be the picture of perfection. But there is no life condition or event that God can't make something or *someone* better as a result. And there is no neighbor whose life is perfect.

Suffering has many different sources, but the healing response is always the same:
- Step into it.
- Get curious.
- Be honest with yourself.
- Be honest with God.
- Unite with the pain of Christ.
- Ask "What is God trying to teach me?"
- How can I make the world better from this experience?
- Choose to love.
- Get up after failing.
- Choose to love again.
- Forgive.
- Find purpose.
- Repeat.

Hope became tangible when I stopped dwelling on myself as damaged and started to wonder what I might learn from all of this. The future of life is unknown. It will bring surprises, confusion, joys, heartbreaks, fears, and sadness. I know God is faithful to His promises because I have witnessed Him outdo my expectations over and over again. He doesn't even know how to fail me, and this realization has provided great peace, even as I prepare to face an array of different challenges yet to come. Healing is not the absence of suffering––but finding suffering's purpose. Joy and mourning can and often do co-exist.

I can choose to let infertility break me. Or I can find the unexpected love story about how it, along with other sufferings, has delivered my greatest joys: the joy of significant spiritual growth, greater strength, increased depth of intimacy with God and my spouse, our beautiful and one-of-a-kind daughter, the hope of another child, the understanding of motherhood as a choice we make daily, and a challenge to uncover my true gifts and purposes. I would not be the woman I am today without my struggles. *Twelve stripes deep––they've made me who I am. Twelve laps on this track, but I still stand.*

And you will, too.

*"Joy is very infectious;
therefore, be always full of joy".*

–Mother Teresa

Acknowledgements

Thank you, Heavenly Father, for your relentless pursuit of me, your impeccable design of woman, your idea of motherhood, and for your incredible creativity and generosity in distributing your gifts and talents to every person you have created.

Thank you, Momma Mary, for your radiant example of motherhood in all of its forms.

Thank you, Pope St. John Paul II and Pope St. Paul VI for sharing such wisdom in clarity *and* charity in your writings.

Thank you, Chris, for your commitment to loving Bella and I so selflessly, and for your undying support of me. I could not have gotten through any of this without you. You are my favorite.

Thank you, Emily, for seeing me! And for contributing this incredible foreword. Your wisdom, encouragement, and honesty has made me better and has truly helped my gifts to flourish. I am so grateful for your friendship, your word magic, and your humor. SIJ.

Thank you, Lisa, for suffering with me and for seeing me as I am! Your support and wisdom have gotten me through some of my toughest days. Your recognition of my value has helped my passions come to life. I am so grateful for your friendship!

Thank you, Julianne, for making me laugh for so many years, for your gift of artistry, for discovering the lotus for me, and for affirming my gifts so frequently. You have helped me to come alive!

Thank you, Jen, for recognizing that I have something important to bring to the table as a Catholic infertile woman and for believing that I could write this book. It was a conversation with you that made me believe I could do it!

Thank you, Melissa V. K., for allowing me to vent and ask so many questions about publishing a book! Your kindness, tips, and wisdom have been invaluable.

Thank you, Chloe, for your kindness and generosity in helping me with so many aspects of getting this book published!

Thank you, Erica, for your guidance in publishing this book! Without your referral to the Killion Group, I would not have been able to push this book out.

Thank you, Stevie, for recognizing my talent in writing this book, for your encouragement, and for helping me to get started.

Thank you, Mom and Dad, for the gift of my Catholic faith, and to Angela as well, for all of your support throughout many surgeries, infertility, and adoption.

Thank you, Bruno Family, for such immense support and encouragement for all the work I do, and for all of your support through surgeries, infertility, and adoption.

Thank you, Ashley, for your friendship, your unwavering support of my passions, and your commitment to improve marriage and family life, and the way our Catholic culture views infertility.

Thank you, Addie, for always being so excited about and interested in my work! Your support has helped my gifts to thrive.

Thank you, Lloyd and Jan Tate, for your incredible contribution to marriages everywhere, for your unwavering support, and for being such good friends to Chris and I.

Thank you, Casey, for suffering with me and for always being willing to listen to the cries of my infertile heart, especially when it was not easy. You are a gem!

Thank you, Lindsey, for seeing me, laughing with me, checking on me when you were aware of so many pregnancy announcements, and sending me that sweet gift after my hysterectomy!

Thank you, Lindsay, for your sweet singing voice, your friendship, and your support throughout the years.

Thank you, Antoniya, for taking such a sweet interest in this book, my story, and our efforts to adopt another child.

Thank you, Dr. Thomas Hilgers, and all those who helped to develop the Creighton Model and NaProTechnology, for your service to women and couples. Thank you to developers and teachers of all fertility awareness based methods!

Thank you, Oscar, Will, and Elise, for recognizing my gift for writing lyrics and rapping, helping me to cultivate it, and for working with me to create some beautiful music.

Thank you, Christopher West, Jennifer Fulwiler, Lloyd and Jan Tate, Anna Saucier, Oscar Rivera, Dr. Naomi Whittaker, Dr. Stephen Hilgers, Chloe Langr, and Bridget Busacker, for your time and generous endorsement of this work that is so important to me. I am so grateful!

Bibliography

1. A D Domar, P C Zuttermeister, R Friedman (1993). "The psychological impact of infertility: a comparison with patients with other medical conditions," Journal of Psychosomatic Obstetrics and Gynaecology. Retrieve from https://pubmed.ncbi.nlm.nih.gov/8142988/.
2. Rachel K Jones (2011). "Beyond Birth Control: The Overlooked Benefits of Oral Contraceptive Pills," Guttmacher Institute. Retrieve from https://www.guttmacher.org/sites/default/files/report_pdf/beyond-birth-control.pdf.
3. IARC Monographs volumes 72, 91 and 100A
4. Larimore, W.L. and Stanford, J.B.: "Post-Fertilization Effects of Oral Contraception and their Relationship to Informed Consent." Arch Fam Med 9: 126-133, 2000.
5. Patrick Yeung, Jr, MD, Shweta Gupta, Sam Gieg (2017). "Endometriosis in Adolescents: A Systematic Review." Journal of Endometriosis and Pelvic Pain Disorders. Retrieve from https://journals.sagepub.com/doi/abs/10.5301/je.5000264.
6. Angelo Stagnaro (2016). "If This is How You Treat Your Friends," National Catholic Register. Retrieve from https://www.ncregister.com/blog/if-this-is-how-you-treat-your-friends.
7. Georgina Chambers, The Conversation (2017.) "Women now have clearer statistics on whether IVF is

likely to work," Medical Press. Retrieve from https://medicalxpress.com/news/2017-07-women-clearer-statistics-ivf-towork.html.

8. Maasburg, L. (2016). Mother Teresa of Calcutta: A Personal Portrait. United States of America: Ignatius Press.

9. Michael E. Gaitley (2016). 33 Days to Morning Glory, A Do-It-Yourself Retreat In Preparation for Marian Consecration. Stockbridge, MA: Marian Press.

10. John Paul II (1984). Apostolic Letter Salvifici Doloris of the Supreme Pontiff John Paul II to the Bishops, to the Priests, to the Religious Families and to the Faithful of the Catholic Church on the Christian Meaning of Human Suffering.

11. Alphonsus Ligouri (1999). The Practice of the Love of Jesus Christ. Missouri: Ligouri Publications.

12. Thomas W. Hilgers (2010). "Near Adhesion-Free Reconstructive Pelvic Surgery: Three Distinct Phases of Progress Over 23 Years." Journal of Gynecologic Surgery.

13. Michael E. Gaitley (2016). Consoling the Heart of Jesus, A Do-It-Yourself Retreat Inspired by the Spiritual Exercises of St. Ignatius. Stockbridge, MA: Marian Press.

14. Zhang J. and Zhang D. (2017). "Prevalence of Tubal Endometriosis." Journal of Minimally Invasive Gynecology. Retrieve from https://www.jmig.org/article/S1553-4650(17)30520-4/pdf.

15. John Paul II (1988). Apostolic Letter Mulieris Dignitatem of the Supreme Pontiff John Paul II on the Dignity and Vocation of Women on the Occasion of the Marian Year.

16. Catechism of the Catholic Church - Latin text copyright (c) Libreria Editrice Vaticana, Citta del Vaticano 1993

17. Jennifer Fulwiler (2020). Your Blue Flame. Michigan: Zondervan Christian Publishing.

Author Bio

Mary grew up right outside of New Orleans, Louisiana, where she grew up loving sports and helping people. This motivated her to acquire her Bachelors of Science in Human Performance and Health Promotion from the University of New Orleans and an Associates in Applied Science as a Physical Therapist Assistant from Delgado. She practiced as a PTA for 6 years. She and Chris got married in 2013 and adopted their daughter, Isabella, in 2016. They live in Mandeville, Louisiana with their golden doodle, and are hoping to adopt again very soon.

Mary is presently a stay/work-at-home mom whose experiences have given her a heart for the infertile and all women of reproductive age in hopes of educating, motivating, and inspiring an appreciation for God's holistic design of woman through fertility awareness. These desires inspired her Taking Back the Terms (now @*whitelotusblooming*) outreach in 2016, to become a Creighton Practitioner in 2018, and to co-found the non-profit, FAbM Base, in 2020, of which she serves as Executive Director.

Mary and her husband were trained as a marriage prep mentor couple in 2018 by Lloyd and Jane Tate and she has spoken about women's health, fertility awareness, and Theology of the Body at various local high schools and parishes for years. She started a personal blog in 2014 and was a columnist for the "Nola Catholic Parenting" section of the Clarion Herald, the Official Newspaper of the Archdiocese of New Orleans for about 3 years. She was featured as one of *Aleteia*'s 7 Catholic women who share about infertility on Instagram and in the *Theology of Home*'s "Daily Collection" for her blog "Infertile, Still Fruitful."

Mary was featured as a speaker at the first virtual *Unexplained Infertility Summit* hosted by Anna Saucier, the *Living Through Infertility Summit* hosted by "Living in the Wait's" Melissa Vande Kieft, and presented two different talks at the *Catholic Link Latin America* Summit. She has been a guest on the *Letters to Women, Mary Kate's, Managing Your Fertility, Charting Towards Intimacy, Engage with Eagle Forum*, and *Natural Misconceptions* podcasts. She co-hosts *The Intersect* podcast with Emily Frase. Learn more and donate to their non-profit at fabmbase.org and find her on IG and FB @WhiteLotusBlooming and @Fabmbase.

CPSIA information can be obtained
at www.ICGtesting.com
Printed in the USA
LVHW050713171022
730843LV00003B/352